MEDICINE'S GRANDEST FRAUD PHD

✳✳✳

DISSERTATION EXPOSING AN ELABORATE 1928 FRAUD AND PERVASIVE IMPACTS ON MODERN MEDICINE & DENTISTRY

by

S. Hale Shakman

Submitted to the Faculty of the American Academy of Biological Dentistry in Fulfillment of the
Requirements for the Degree of Doctor of Philosophy in the History of Dentistry
"Medicine's Grandest Fraud –Revelations of a Critical Review of Dentistry in the 20th Century"
July 1999

INSTITUTE OF SCIENCE
www.InstituteOfScience.com

INSTITUTE OF SCIENCE
InstituteOfScience.com
mail@InstituteOfScience.com

First Printed 1998 (Parts I & II); Augmented 1999 (Part III)
Complete work first printed 29 February 2004
Reprinted 2010

Warning and Disclaimer: Although every possible effort has been
made to assure the accuracy and correctness of information herein,
the publisher hereby: apologizes and disclaims liability for any
errors which have escaped editing; and disclaims any and all
dental, medical or legal liability in the event the contents of
this book are utilized as a direct source of any dental or medical
advice. The reader is encouraged to access original works
discussed herein to assure accuracy of information, and to refer
any medical questions concerning discussions herein and related
dental or medical treatment to appropriate professionals. A proper
professional assessment of all of a person's medical conditions
must always be taken into account prior to development of a
treatment plan. In this regard, as differing professional opinions
abound, a "second opinion" (or more) is highly recommended.

The AUTOMED Project:
- *AUTOHEMOTHERAPY REFERENCE MANUAL*
- *REFERENCE MANUAL ROSENOW ET AL*
- ***MEDICINE'S GRANDEST FRAUD PHD***

Printed in the United States of America

$$* \quad * \quad *$$

DEDICATION – To Edward Arana, DDS

This publication is dedicated to the memory of Edward Arana, DDS, founding President of the American Academy of Biological Dentistry, and prominent if not preeminent modern pioneer in promoting awareness of the connection between oral and systemic diseases.

The writer is particularly indebted to Dr. Arana for his courageous championing of the definitive work by Martin Fischer, M.D., *Death and Dentistry*, 1940, prominently featured in Part III, Section 5, herein. Dr. Arana gave me a copy of the Fischer book on the occasion of our first meeting, and demanded I read it.

I had previously been only slightly familiar with the Fischer book, but soon came to realize that it exhaustively validated and augmented the works of E.C. Rosenow, the subject of my own prior and continuing long study, also as seen herein -- which of course is why Dr. Arana shared it with me with such urgency.

Although he had already been impaired by a stroke prior to our first meeting, Dr. Arana's powerful intellect and vision beamed forth from his big brain through his sparkling magical eyes, as he shared this compelling and delightful perspective with me in our every meeting. His mind and vision were clear and unrivaled relative to the challenge, opportunity, and even responsibility facing dentists and dentistry as the world moves into a new millennium. I am forever grateful for and inspired by his spirit, support and friendship.

S. H. Shakman, 29 February 2004.

TABLE OF CONTENTS

               * * * * * *

IMPACT ON THE HISTORY OF DENTISTRY

TABLES, EXHIBITS, FIGURES

ABOUT THE AUTHOR

AUTHOR BIOGRAPHICAL SKETCH

     S. Hale Shakman has been involved with analysis of health and related programs since 1966-9, when he served with the U.S. State Department's Agency for International Development (A.I.D.) in Washington, D.C. As Program Officer for the Vietnam Program's Public Health Sector, he participated in the overall planning, development and coordination of both direct assistance and training efforts, including oversight of American Medical Association and American Dental Association education contracts, assessments of health facility and construction needs, and coordination with U.S. military and other free world contributors. This included two temporary assignments to Vietnam totaling 5 months, and a Meritorious Service award. He subsequently served in a program management capacity at the Office of Economic Opportunity in Washington, D.C.
     Shakman left government service to accept the position of Deputy Director of International Programs (Operations) for the Pathfinder Fund, a private non profit population and health service organization. Later, as an independent consultant and writer, he assisted Maryland, Washington State and Alaska in developing Administration on Aging sponsored nutrition programs; researched, designed and wrote the Planning and Operations Guide for the National Summer Youth Sports Program (sponsored by the President's Council on Physical Fitness and the N.C.A.A.); designed an information system to serve disabled children in the Headstart Program; and compiled and edited THE BLACK PAGES Directory and Resource Guide for People of Color Publications of San Francisco. Additional publications include articles in USA TODAY and the British journal Nature.
     Following graduation from Northwestern University (BA), Shakman was accepted into Georgetown University Graduate School's direct to PhD program in History of Political Thought, earning honors and election to Pi Sigma Alpha honor society. He withdrew with permission from Georgetown to accept temporary assignment to Vietnam for the U.S. Department of State. He was subsequently a participant in the Scholars' Colloquium at the Library of Congress, and resumed and completed his PhD program requirements in History of Dentistry by special petition through the American Academy of Biological Dentistry. This current publication, *MEDICINE'S GRANDEST FRAUD PHD*, comprises his Dissertation.
     Shakman is Executive Director of the Institute of Science in Santa Monica, California.

PREFACE

The idea that diseases of the teeth might contribute to or even
cause various systemic diseases has been discussed from at least as
early as the 7th Century B.C. up to the present. This concept,
known as the concept of "focal infection", reached a high level of
prominence and sophistication in the first part of the Twentieth
Century following the particularly well-publicized works of William
Hunter of England. But despite the conclusively-refining studies
of Edward C. Rosenow, in association with former A.M.A. Presidents
Frank Billings and Charles Mayo, plus Weston Price, Russell Haden
and many others, the concept of focal infection has been playing
"Rip van Winkle" for the past half-century.
The writer first stumbled across E. C. Rosenow (and subsequently
through him the focal infection concept) in a 1915 article by C.H.
Pierce on autogenous vaccine therapy. In his discussions, Pierce
invoked the accomplishments of immunology greats Koch and Ehrlich,
and in a culminatory breath, lavishly praised an E. C. Rosenow; but
he made absolutely no reference to the generally-acknowledged
originator of autogenous-vaccine-therapy, Sir Almroth Wright. Who
was this E. C. Rosenow?
The works of Sir Almroth E. Wright on autogenous vaccines are
truly legendary, as immortalized in G. Bernard Shaw's *Doctor's
Dilemma*. Shaw's Dr. Ridgeon was a master of autogenous vaccines,
and spoke of "opsonins", the sticky stuff in blood that stuck to
"invaders" like tasty butter on bland bread, setting up the
invaders for consumption by the phagocytes, turning those blind,
docile blobs of protoplasm (the phagocytes) into efficient killer-
"pac-men". This was Sir Almroth Wright, introduced as such by
Shaw, the real-life inventor of autogenous vaccines and "opsonins".
 So who was Rosenow?
And how in 1915, with Wright still a very vital force in
medicine, and yet a score away from weaseling the London Times into
setting up Arthur Fleming for a piece of a Nobel that could as
easily have gone to a janitor. Wright, the unquestioned moving
force behind autogenous vaccines and opsonins. Sir "Almost Right"
to his detractors, and one of the immortal founding fathers of
immunology to supporters like Ivan Roitt, originator of the
"autoimmunity" craze of recent years .... the one and the only Sir
Almroth E. Wright. So who was Rosenow?

It turns out that, by the end of 1915, Rosenow had already
published more than 70 articles in the mainstream medical
literature, including a landmark 1915 *JAMA* summary article which
showed how bacteria from infected "oral foci" of humans with
various diseases (e.g. arthritis, appendicitis, stomach ulcers,
etc.) would "electively locate" in corresponding organs of
laboratory animals. Rosenow was to solidify and expand on this
work over the next four decades, three of them as the Mayo Clinic's
Head of Experimental Bacteriology. By every test available to
medical science, plus some he invented; and verified and sworn to
by numerous unimpeachable medical authorities; Rosenow seemed to

have found what modern science continues to search for -- an environmental (bacterial) cause for various degenerative diseases in so-called "constitutionally-" or "genetically-predisposed" persons. Yet on further examination it appeared that, to the extent his work was not being ignored, it was maligned and generally thought to have been disproved.

A review of literature critical of Rosenow's work, and underlying references, was undertaken in an attempt to determine what had happened to him; this review disclosed common and indispensable reference to a 1928 article by W. L. Holman, which had portrayed Rosenow's 1915 data as inconclusive. On examination, it was found that Holman had perpetrated a clever but nonetheless blatant deception - one whose spectacular ramifications might hardly have been imagined, even by its author.

In the first instance and most essentially, this work fully exposes details of Holman's carefully constructed 1928 fabrication. Secondly, it reviews the incredible fashion in which it has come to assert a major and continuing influence on the history and development of modern dentistry and medicine. Holman's handiwork comprises the key and indispensable foundation for layers of subsequent denial of the importance of, and general disregard for the revolutionary works of Rosenow and associates as well as for the venerable concept of focal infection in general. Holman's deception thus continues to comprise the fraudulent foundation on which rests an inverted pyramid of ignorance and unnecessary speculation as to the cause of a range of human diseases. (See <3> THE FACTS).

At the same time, Holman's deception appears to be the indispensable foundational "scientific" justification for the practice of treating and filling infected root-canals, so called "root-canal therapy" or "endodontics" (*endo* - inside, *dontics* - teeth). This is because Holman, while not specifically dealing with treated root-canals, did deal with Rosenow's results for various oral foci. These included so-called "devitalized" teeth, i.e., teeth which and whose roots are no longer alive, i.e., including all root-canal-treated teeth. But the connection is not simply so indirect.

And the endodontics literature has since served as the unquestionable primary driving force that has perpetuated the impact of Holman's fraud, as shown in this study, although there is no indication that Holman's handiwork has previously been exposed or acknowledged to be fraudulent. A chronology of events that reflect this inescapable conclusion is presented in Appendix E: A "CON" CHRON.

Then seemingly like a cancerous organ within the developing body of dentistry, the intrinsically flawed and deadly concept of "root canal therapy" gained full acceptance and full integration into common modern dental practice. And the kind and cooperative body of medicine went along.

But the full story is insidiously much deeper than just Holman's fraud and its perpetuation (albeit apparently unwittingly) by root-canal "therapy" advocates.

Guided by some particularly relevant observations of George Meinig, D.D.S., a founding member of the American Association of Endodontists a half century ago and recent author of the book *Root Canal Cover-up*, the writer was impelled to search for information which might shed additional light on what had occurred and why.

In conversation with the writer, Dr. Meinig had mentioned the issue of large doses of bacteria given to animals by Rosenow as being fundamental in continuing anti-Rosenow sentiment. Insofar as the writer's notes included reference to this argument by Louis I. Grossman, D.D.S., a search for added historical information on Grossman was initiated. This has been incorporated herein as APPENDIX F - THE GROSSMAN FILE.

That opposition to Rosenow and focal infection did not originate with Grossman, or Holman, is clearly evident in the existence of even earlier focal-infection critics, e.g. Percy Howe (1919), John P. Buckley, and others mentioned by Meinig in his book as having been particularly vocal and important (plus others as discussed in APPENDICES E and G). On this question, of particular interest to this writer were two references by Louis Grossman to editorials in the *Journal of the A.D.A.*. One in 1938 was cited as pivotal in the history of endodontics, and reference to another from 1935 seemed to misrepresent the position of Hunter early in the century. Both were written by early *J.A.D.A.* Editor C.N. Johnson. Thus it was back into the library to review the editorial pages of the *J.A.D.A.* in its early years. Notes from this foray are incorporated into APPENDIX G - *J.A.D.A.* - THE EARLY YEARS.

C. N. Johnson is high on the list of persons contributing to the current (deplorable) state of affairs. Johnson was President of the American Dental Association in 1924-5 and Editor of JADA from 1925 to the time of his death in 1938. Some of his key writings and editorials during this period are featured in APPENDIX G.

It turns out that Johnson was Dean of the dental school in Chicago which Meinig attended (The Chicago College of Dental Surgery, which became Loyola Dental in the year in Meinig's senior year). According to Meinig, Johnson was an expert, probably the best, in the use of gold foil as a filling material; and "a great guy". This may help understand, in part, how we got to where we are today.

We may view C.N. Johnson an enthusiastic artist of the mouth, performing beautiful, intricate work that was also practical -- it allowed his patients to use their teeth. At the time of the onset of popularization of the focal infection concept, Johnson was in his prime. He truly believed he was doing work that was of benefit to his patients, which it was, and he was the best. Was he now to cease doing this work, merely because some upstart bacteriologists claimed that down the road these teeth would cause disease?

Johnson repeatedly returned to the theme of the value of clinical experience, in preference to the uncertainty of bacteriological work, and to the dentist's expert knowledge of teeth compared to the cursory, minimal knowledge of physicians.

The field of dentistry, as exemplified in Johnson's work, evolved from primary emphasis on the technical side, and secondarily became concerned with scientific and systemic implications. This seems to still be the case, probably necessarily so. There is an inherent conflict of interest between the objective of "saving teeth" and the investigation of whether teeth can be saved. With all due respect to the legions of well-intentioned hard-working dentists in the world, the total relegation to dentistry of decision-making concerning pulp-involved or otherwise infected teeth is clearly a case of "the fox in the chicken coop". This is not to say that even a single dentist has ever retained a single tooth that was known to be harmful; this is saying that it is extremely difficult if not impossible for sworn tooth-savers to be totally objective on this issue.

The overall picture that emerges is one that does not reflect particularly well on the concept of dentistry as it has evolved into modern practice. It seems clear that root-involved teeth are doomed and must be extracted, the sooner the better. Additionally, in the case of pulpless or other infected teeth that had remained in the mouth for a long time, or in areas of previous extractions (including, e.g., "wisdom teeth"), the added complication of residual bone infections must also be addressed.

The question then is at what point in the pre-root-involvement stage is the tooth doomed in any case? In the case of deep fillings in place over a long period of time, the likelihood of invasion of the root is ever increasing. As Henrici and Hartzell 1919 have pointed out and no one has ever refuted (see APPENDIX D - THE STERILITY ISSUE), the invasion of the root from either caries or pyorrhea is a long drawn-out process. Once infection from caries has gained access to the dentinal tubules, is there any way to stop the gradual, apparently inexorable movement toward the pulp? Is there any type of procedure that can actually do this? If not, the implication of futility of attempting to "save" such teeth seems clear.

Future investigations of this problem must incorporate the requisite methods of Rosenow, as verified by Price, Billings, Mayo, Haden and others, so as to assure that we are not wasting our time and resources. In the meanwhile, insofar as there is so much evidence against the retention of suspect teeth, are they to be allowed to remain? Alternatively, would it not be preferable to use laboratory animals (rather than humans) in experimentation to determine if _any_ compromised teeth are safe to retain?

Of course, efforts must be ever- increased against the onset of oral infection; as Drs. Meinig, Weston Price and many others have pointed out, this must involve some means of curtailing exposure to conditions that contribute to it. Say goodbye to white flour and sugar, for openers.

So far we have been discussing dentistry, and the implications of this work on the highly trained and committed persons who have dedicated their lives to this arena.

How about the field of medicine? We must not forget that the effects of the situation are not confined to dentists and their patients, but rather that the ramifications for medicine are quite major. We are reminded that the best and brightest of the medical world, the pride of the American Medical Association in the first half of the century, have been maligned by these events, to some extent discredited and defamed, and certainly ignored.

Frank Billings was President of the AMA just after the turn of the century, and is acknowledged by some as the father of American medical education. To Billings, the high point of his professional career was his Lane Lecture Series presentation on focal infection in 1915, which showcased for the world the dramatic results of animal experimentation by E. C. Rosenow and associates. Was he just taken in by Rosenow, with whom he had worked closely for 12 years on the subject?

And how about Rosenow? Following this 12-year research stint with Billings and Hektoen, etc. Rosenow served for nearly three decades with the Mayo Foundation as head of experimental bacteriology - from 1915-1944, then moved to the California Institute of Technology after retirement from Mayo, and continued working and publishing through 1958. Was he faking it? Could he possibly have fooled everyone at Mayo, etc., for all that time? Of course not.

Then there's Charles Mayo, particularly well known for his intellectual prowess. Mayo was also an AMA President - and nobody's fool.

And Walter Bierring, President of the AMA in 1934, who predicted in JAMA in 1938 that Rosenow's work would come to be regarded as "medical guide of the future". Was he duped too?

Truly the justifiably proud tradition of the American Medical Association has been subverted; at some point medicine must reclaim this tradition and those prerogatives relating to the investigation of disease causation that have been usurped by historical events described in this report. Nor can medicine fully evade proper criticism of its gross abdication of responsibility of one part of the body, the mouth, to the separate jurisdiction of dentistry.

And at the bottom line is the fact that there are the millions of persons who are unnecessarily suffering from a range of ailments known to be secondary to oral foci.

Yes, clearly there is much more at stake here than may first appear, much more than merely the issue of root canal "therapy". But at the heart of the problem is this very issue, this oxymoron that might be better be referred to as root-canal "sepsis"; root canal "therapy" -- the practice whose whose formal name "endodontics" purports to reflect knowledge of the inside of teeth and whose reality reflects an organized commitment to discredit any (many) facts which indicate root canal "therapy" is anything but

therapeutic; root-canal-"therapy", a.k.a. endodontics -- terms
which may come to be regarded as the ultimate in quackery.

   Finally, a word of particular thanks to George Meinig, D.D.S.,
F.A.C.D. and Christopher J. Hussar, D.D.S., D.O., Edward Arana,
D.D.S. of the American Academy of Biological Dentistry, and a
number of their fine associates for their gracious welcome and
encouragement. And to Cecil H. Uyehara, the writer's mentor in the
U.S. Dept. of State three decades ago, who imparted the confidence
to tackle a project such as this. And to dear family members whose
unflagging support over the years has been essential and
indispensable.

   Nonetheless the writer retains full responsibility for any and
all statements made herein, as well as for the "rough" condition of
this work, to be improved as possible and hopefully utilized in the
meantime. Thank you, the reader, for your kind understanding.

                    S. H. Shakman   7 March 1998

Part I: *Doctoring the Numbers: Medicine's Greatest Fraud*

<1> BRIEF REVIEWS OF FOCAL INFECTION AND DENTISTRY

A. OVERVIEW OF THE HISTORY OF THE CONCEPT OF FOCAL INFECTION

   The concept of focal infection dates back to the earliest times in recorded medical history. In the 7th Century B.C., when King Ashurbanipal of Assyria criticized his physician for failing to cure the king's rheumatism, the physician wrote a stinging retort in which it was asserted that the cause of the king's problems was in his diseased mouth.

   Reference is commonly made to Hippocrates's subsequent mention of the subject, although this was not particularly emphasized by him or his associates. But it was there.

   The impetus for greater attention to the problem in modern times seems clearly related to Benjamin Rush's activism on the subject. Rush, a signer of the Declaration of Independence, was the most prominent physician of his time. His favorable reputation unquestionably developed as a result of having greatly relieved the severe arthritic symptoms of most of those patients who followed his advice to have their diseased teeth removed. Within two months nearly all of a number of former crippled persons no longer needed their crutches. Rush himself emphasized that his work merely substantiated that which was common knowledge among health practitioners.

   A number of articles were written on the subject through the 19th Century, including several on the relation between eye diseases and diseased teeth, as compiled by A.D. Black in 1915. But the major force propelling knowledge of the subject into the modern era was the work of William Hunter of England at the turn of the century.

   Soon afterwards, and concurrent with much of Hunter's well-publicized activity during the early years of the century, Frank Billings of Chicago became involved in researching this situation in a major way. Billings had served at the very start of the century as President of the AMA, and was well known as essentially the founding father of modern medical education. But following his stint as AMA President, Billings's attention was largely focused on the problem of oral focal infection. In close cooperation with Ludwig Hektoen, Charles Mayo and other renowned researchers, Billings was most ably assisted by the able bacteriological work of a young and brilliant Edward C. Rosenow.

   In 1915 Billings presented a major lecture series at Stanford U. on the subject of focal infection, the Lane Lecture Series. Billings referred to studies conducted over the course of more than a decade as concrete evidence of the truth of the concept of focal infection. This included data showing how, using Rosenow's carefully developed culture procedures, different specific human diseases could be replicated in laboratory animals.

   In modern times of mass communication, this work would be widely touted as having proved causation of these diseases in accord with the venerable Koch-Henle criteria; indeed, for some years afterward, the medical world generally accepted and began to implement the implicated course of action. This necessarily involved the extraction of diseased teeth, insofar as it had been proved that they comprised nests from which harmful organisms emanated and caused all of the various, chronic, mysterious diseases.

But then something(s) happened that seemed to discredit this work. Of course, there was resistance all along, for the application of knowledge following from the work of Billings, Rosenow, Mayo, Price, Haden, Austin, and many of their associates, as cited herein, basically meant that modern dentistry had to shut down. Yes, it meant and still means that modern dentistry is a mistake, and not a healing art. Rather it can be clearly shown that modern dentistry, the whole darn concept and practice, is probably the most harmful fad in the history of humanity.

The major factor in the ascendance and continued propping up of modern dentistry, to the detriment of medical science and human health, is an insidiously fraudulent article that has successfully fooled all of dentistry as well as medicine. The article was written by an apparently jealous rival of Rosenow, W.L. Holman. As we will revisit in a later section of this work, Holman had been after Rosenow since as early as 1914, attacking him first on his breakthrough work on the subject of bacteriological mutations. But when Holman in 1927-8 took on Rosenow's work on focal infection, and thereby Rosenow's case against dentistry, Holman gained an organized group of vitally-involved supporters. Advocates of root-canal "therapy" and dentistry in general were anxiously receptive to citing statistics refuting Rosenow. That Holman's statistics were nothing but a sham, a blatant fraud, will be clearly demonstrated herein. But both factors were needed. Holman's fraud could not have gained so deep and broad a following without its adoption by the dentists, who do not seem to have recognized it as fraudulent. And it may not have been possible for the dentists to have presented so solid a front, or otherwise even gotten near the strength needed to challenge Rosenow, without the coalescing and convincing construction of Holman.

B. A BRIEF HISTORY OF DENTISTRY, OR DENTISTRY'S BRIEF HISTORY

A form of jaw surgery was practiced in England during the Stone Age, apparently associated with abscesses at the roots of teeth. Although caries were still uncommon, the problem of jaw abscesses seems to have been common for Europeans and North Africans of the New Stone Age. Dentists of the time would drive the tooth sideways, and then pull it. Over time, probe like instruments were developed to aid in tooth extraction, which practice virtually comprised dentistry through medieval times.

According to Sharp 1937, Bourdet was extirpating pulps and filling roots of anterior teeth with gold as early as 1757. Following this, in the late 18th century and through the 19th, the mentality concerning dentistry was largely shaped by John Hunter (1728-93), perhaps the most influential scientist of his time and friend and mentor to Edward Jenner. John Hunter, best known for his work on comparative anatomy, had advocated the complete removal of dental pulps before fillings were inserted into cavities, a practice which remained popular even into the early 20th century.

Up through nearly the mid-19th century, dentistry was a trade passed from dentist to dentist. In 1838, Horace Hayden founded the Baltimore College of Dental Surgery, the first dental school in the world. And while several states began requiring the registration of dentists as early as 1868, it was not until 1900 that this was required in all the states. Thus did the United States give birth to the field of dentistry, which has now been exported to the rest of the world.

<2> TRUST AND FRAUD IN SCIENCE

THE IMPORTANCE OF TRUST IN SCIENCE

   "The scientific research enterprise is built on a foundation of
trust: trust that the results reported by others are valid. ..."
[Alberts A & K Shine, <u>Science</u> 266, 1994, 1660]

   Here's a new twist. How about falsely discrediting someone's
valid results, and then having a whole church built on that false
discreditation. Sounds a bit complicated, and who cares anyway?
   How about if that church is modern dentistry, and by extension,
modern medicine? A little extreme? Please read on, because this
story is absolutely true, and it probably affects you.

FRAUD IN SCIENCE - THE BIG ONE; YOU <u>CAN</u> FOOL ALL THE PEOPLE

   It seems so unlikely, so impossible, that anyone could have
successfully executed so embarrassingly ludicrous and long-lived a
fraud as Holman's Deception of 1927-8, which involved the mis-
manipulation of data to discredit research results which (a) could
not and still cannot be refuted and (b) have otherwise been
repeatedly confirmed experimentally. Nonetheless, Holman's
Deception continues to play a decisive role in the denial of
indispensable information to modern medicine and dentistry, thereby
contributing to the needless suffering and early demise of
millions, insidiously and persistently infecting the literature of
medicine and dentistry like a modern computer "virus" -- yes, there
is a terrible "virus" loose in the history of medicine and
dentistry, and it's time to expose it and eradicate it.

   The sad truth is that correcting the literature will be no simple
task, as implications on medicine and dentistry in general are
major and pervasive, and in the case of one field, "endodontics",
terminal. As drastic as this sounds, in a sense it may be an
understatement -- the terminally implicated field may not be merely
"endodontics" (a.k.a. root-canal-therapy) but rather the whole of
modern dentistry.

   Holman's action, if not an innocent, extremely stupid and even
laughable error, was an outright fraud. But Holman clearly was not
an imbecile; the detail of his data manipulation discloses
unquestionable, albeit insidious, talent. This coupled with his
willful exclusion of meaningful factual data clearly establishes
that his essential contribution to the history of medicine
comprises its greatest fraud ever.

<3> THE FACTS

A FRAUD HAS BEEN PERPETRATED
    The modern scientific literature commonly refers to similarities
between such diseases as multiple sclerosis, arthritis, diabetes,
and thyroiditis "in genetically predisposed individuals", such as
"characteristic inflammatory destructive lesions" [Waksman 1989] or
hypothesized involvement of an "auto-immune" mechanism. In the
earlier part of the 20th Century, the grouping of these diseases as
similar was commonly associated with E.C. Rosenow and his works
which appeared to have established a common bacterial cause.
    Early in his career, E. C. Rosenow worked closely with Frank
Billings, building on the works of William Hunter, Mayo and
Billings on oral infection, and the works of Sir Almroth Wright on
autogenous vaccines. Over an active professional career spanning
more than five decades, Rosenow conducted extensive series of
animal experiments and other tests which supported the concept of
elective localization of bacteria or their toxins (emanating from
oral foci and carried through the bloodstream) as a factor in
diverse diseases; see list of disease conditions addressed by
Rosenow, APPENDIX A.
    In 1915, Rosenow's initial summary report of animal experiments
over the previous twelve years was published in the *Journal of the
A.M.A.*, and elegantly showcased by former AMA President Frank
Billings in his Lane Lecture Series presentation. This work was
regarded by Billings as the high point of his already illustrious
career. Building on this solid base, Rosenow went on to serve
nearly three decades with the Mayo Foundation.
    In 1928 W. L. Holman challenged Rosenow's well-publicized and
generally accepted 1915 report with a claimed "rearrangement of
Rosenow's data". This challenge over time has come to assume
pivotal importance as a common and key reference in literature
underlying the modern relationship between medicine and dentistry
(e.g., see Figure 1 and APPENDIX C: "HOLMAN'S LEGACY - A CON
CHRON"), and beyond that, to have had a profound negating effect on
progress which had been made by Rosenow and others pertaining to
the cause, prevention and treatment of a number of disease
conditions that continue to plague mankind.
    In fact, Holman's rearrangement is a cleverly designed deception
which neither refuted nor even substantively challenged Rosenow's
actual results; rather, it diverted the reader to selective and
essentially meaningless information.
    For example, as listed in Exhibit 1, Rosenow reported stomach or
duodenum hemorrhages developed in 60% of 103 laboratory animals
injected with bacteria (as isolated) from stomach ulcer patients;
compared to smaller percentages of animals injected with bacteria
from patients with other diseases. Rosenow's data was presented in
the following form:

Lesions with stomach or duodenum hemorrhages developed in:
60% of 103 injected with bacteria from stomach ulcer patients;
versus

```
 6% of 68 injected with bacteria from appendicitis,
29% of 41     "       "       "       "   cholecystitis,
23% of 71     "       "       "       "   rheumatic fever,
10% of 20     "       "       "       "   erythema nodosom,
29% of 61     "       "       "       "   herpes zoster,
21% of 19     "       "       "       "   mumps,
 4% of 40     "       "       "       "   myositis,
 7% of 44     "       "       "       "   myocarditis, and
17% of 41     "       "       "       "   miscellaneous patients.
```

Overall, there was a far greater likelihood (about four times on average) that the strain from stomach ulcers would cause stomach ulcers in laboratory animals, as compared with strains from any of these other conditions.

Holman multiplied each of the above percentages by respective numbers, calculating from Rosenow's data that lesions-in-the-stomach-with-hemorrhages had developed in 62 (60% of the 103) animals injected with bacteria from stomach ulcer patients; vs. 4 (6% of 68) animals injected with appendicitis-associated bacteria, 12 (29% of 41), cholecystitis, 16 (23% of 71) rheumatic fever, etc., for each of items. Holman then summed all of these "others", totalling 68 of 405 animals injected with bacteria from other-than-stomach-ulcer patients.

Holman added the "62" and "68" (ignoring the fact it was 62 of 103; v. 68 of 405) to derive a total of 130 animals with stomach lesions; and exhibited the values "62" and "68" as percentages (48% and 52%) of the 130 animals with stomach lesions with hemorrhages. He made absolutely no reference at all to the fact that a much smaller number of animals had been injected with bacteria from stomach ulcer patients (105) than from other patients (405)! This was the basis for Holman's carefully worded ("weasel-worded") statement "that it is roughly a 50 per cent chance whether any particular localization occurs with a 'specific' or 'non-specific' strain". Then, based on this faulty and essentially meaningless construction, he issued the improperly consequent and false claim that "the specificity of bacteria involved has not been proved".

Holman himself performed no experiments. He simply manipulated Rosenow's data in this fashion, and based his pre-determined anti-Rosenow conclusion on this faulty perspective.

Incredible! Beyond incredible! He got away with it, and he is still getting away with it. And you and/or your loved ones are, or will be, his victims.

Table 1 provides a summary of Rosenow's results as manipulated by Holman's handiwork. To ease initial comparison, Table 1 lists only one of Rosenow's three categories of bacteria, the "when isolated" category. (Table 1a exhibits the full detail, including bacteria "when isolated", "later", and "after animal passage".)

Exhibits 1 and 2 are photocopies of the original tables in Rosenow 1915 and Holman 1928. At first, second and even third glance, the two Exhibits do not appear to refer to the same information, so complete is the maltransformation by Holman.

We may readily conclude that Holman's action was not one of ignorance by:

(1) the level of detail to which Holman went in deriving his calculations - for example to come up with the number "68" above he had to calculate numbers injected for each of the above disease-associated percentages, and then total them; derive the "62"; add "62" plus "68"; and then calculate them as percentages of a total 130; i.e., 13 separate calculations for just this one phony "48% to 52%" comparison (all this without a hand calculator). And in that Holman displays some 36 sets of so-derived calculations, it was necessary for him to have undertaken hundreds of separate calculations in deriving his "rearrangement". Not that they were particularly difficult; rather this clearly shows the man had a plan, and that plan was to deceive his medical colleagues; in retrospect it may be offered that he clearly succeeded, at least as of the current time, probably far beyond his wildest expectations.

(2) the purposeful omission by Holman of reference to total numbers of animals injected by type, as reflected in Table 1. For example in the above-illustrated case concerning stomach lesions with hemorrhages (with bacteria "when isolated", the only meaningful comparison would involve 60% (62 of 103) v. an average of 17% (68 of 405), or a three-and-a-half times greater incidence of bacteria from patients with stomach ulcers causing ulcers with hemorrhages in the experimental animals.

(3) Holman's careful wording of his reference to his deceptive presentation. His "50% chance" wording was precise and technically correct, but his "rearranged" data were meaningless, and his statement that "the specificity of bacteria involved has not been proved" is groundless (other than based on nonsense) and in fact false.

In 1940 Rosenow published results of more extensive series of experiments by himself, eleven co-workers and 20 others, involving more than 11,000 animals. As shown in Table 2, these studies overwhelmingly confirmed Rosenow's earlier results.

Again, it must be emphasized that the only data presented by Holman was that contained in the last two columns of Tables 1 and 1a. Substantively the Holman "data" is meaningless. Its only purpose was to purposefully deceive.

CONSERVATIVE NATURE OF ROSENOW'S RESULTS [Rosenow 1934]:

Beyond the mere statistical correction provided through exposure of the dastardly deception of Holman, the situation is even more skewed in favor of Rosenow (as will unquestionably be once again confirmed when his experiments are replicated by some discerning modern laboratory). In reporting his results, Rosenow had leaned consistently toward understatement: "The statistical representation of specific effects obtained in experiments on animals, ... striking as it is, does not represent adequately the findings noted at necropsy. Following the injection organs of the animals corresponding to the organs from which the strains were derived were often much more pronounced than were those in similar structures following injection of strains from other sources. The value ... of a small hemorrhage in or around one joint, or of slightly turbid joint fluid, following injection of a strain obtained in a case other than arthritis, is as great as one or more greatly swollen joints, with numerable hemorrhages, containing markedly turbid joint fluid, such as commonly follows injection of a strain obtained in a case of arthritis."

Table 1: ROSENOW'S (1916) RESULTS* VS HOLMAN'S (1928) "REARRANGEMENT"**
          (with bacteria "as isolated"; see Table 1a for full details)

| LESIONS IN ANIMALS': | SOURCE OF STRAIN; PATIENTS WITH: | Rosenow's Data | | Holman's Portrayal |
		ANIMALS INJECTED	% WITH LESIONS	NUMBER W/LES.
Joints	Rheumatic fever	71	66%	(= 47) 36%
	***Other diseases	437	19%	(= 84) 64
				131
Endocardium	Endocarditis	44	84%	(= 37) 30%
	Rheumatic fever	71	46%	(= 33) 27%
	***Other diseases	393	13%	(= 52) 42%
				122
Myocardium	Rheumatic fever	71	44%	(= 32) 38%
	Myositis	40	35%	(= 14) 17%
	***Other diseases	397	9%	(= 36) 44%
				82
Muscles	Rheumatic fever	71	27%	(= 19) 24%
	Myositis	40	75%	(= 30) 38%
	***Other diseases	397	7%	(= 29) 37%
				78
Stomach/ Duodenum (w/hemorr.)	Stomach ulcer	103	60%	(= 62) 48%
	***Other diseases	405	17%	(= 68) 52%
				130
Stomach/ Duodenum (w/ulcer)	Stomach ulcer	103	60%	(= 62) 67%
	***Other diseases	405	7%	(= 30) 33%
				92
Gallbladder	Cholecystitis	41	80%	(= 33) 43%
	***Other diseases	467	9%	(= 43) 57%
				76
Appendix	Appendicitis	68	68%	(= 46) 71%
	***Other diseases	440	4%	(= 19) 29%
				65
Kidneys	Rheumatic fever	71	39%	(= 28) 52%
	***Other diseases	437	6%	(= 26) 48%
				54
Skin	Erythema nodosum	20	90%	Not listed
	Herpes zoster	61	70%	by Holman
	***Other diseases	427	4%	
Parotid	Mumps	19	73%	Not listed
	***Other diseases	489	0%	by Holman
Pancreas	Mumps	19	42%	Not listed
	***Other diseases	489	4%	by Holman

EXHIBIT A: PHOTOCOPY: ROSENOW'S 1915 DATA

Rosenow, E. C., J.A.M.A. LXV, 1688 (1915).

ELECTIVE LOCALIZATION OF STREPTOCOCCI

Source of Streptococci		Strains (220)	Animals Injected (533)	Percentage of Animals Showing Lesions in																	
				Appendix	Stomach Hemor.	Stomach Ulcer	Duodenum	Gallbladder	Pancreas	Intestines	Joints	Endocardium	Pericardium	Myocardium	Muscles	Kidney	Lung	Skin	Tongue	Eye	Parotid
Appendicitis	When isolated	14	68	58	6	1	1	0	9	29	21	0	9	12	0	0	0	0	3	0
	Later	8	26	15	19	15	4	0	0	22	19	0	12	23	0	0	0	0	0	0
	After animal passage	7	22	45	45	36	40	0	20	36	20	0	20	25	18	0	0	0	0	0
Ulcer of stomach in man	When isolated	18	103	2	50	60	20	3	7	16	12	4	5	0	5	0	0	0	0	0
	Later	8	22	5	5	0	5	0	0	18	14	0	0	0	0	0	0	0	0	0
	After animal passage	7	39	0	23	33	30	15	15	21	5	0	3	3	8	15	0	0	0	0
Cholecystitis	When isolated	12	41	6	29	15	80	5	17	17	19	0	2	7	5	5	2	0	0	0
	Later	5	14	14	28	14	7	0	0	21	14	0	0	0	7	0	0	0	0	0
	After animal passage	4	16	0	31	13	56	19	13	25	19	0	12	0	12	6	0	0	0	0
Rheumatic fever	When isolated	24	71	8	23	18	3	3	13	66	46	27	44	27	39	4	0	0	10	0
	Later	8	14	0	14	21	0	0	0	21	21	0	28	0	21	0	0	0	0	0
	After animal passage	5	19	21	37	21	5	21	0	37	53	32	37	16	42	21	0	0	11	0
Erythema nodosum	When isolated	6	29	0	10	0	0	0	5	20	20	10	0	35	10	5	80	0	5	0
	Later	3	9	0	22	0	11	0	0	11	11	0	0	0	0	0	22	0	0	0
	After animal passage	6	14	0	21	0	50	0	7	50	14	7	14	50	7	43	43	0	0	0
Herpes zoster	When isolated	11	61	10	29	8	16	2	8	11	5	11	5	11	5	21	70	15	15	0
	Later	6	15	0	13	7	7	13	7	40	7	0	20	40	7	20	7	0	13	0
	After animal passage	4	7	0	28	10	0	0	0	43	0	14	0	28	0	43	28	14	0	0
Mumps	When isolated	9	19	15	21	5	21	42	10	42	15	0	37	3	5	15	15	0	0	73
	Later	5	8	12	0	0	0	12	12	24	24	0	12	12	0	12	12	0	0	24
Myositis	When isolated	3	40	2	4	10	2	7	7	20	10	0	35	75	2	0	7	0	8	0
Endocarditis	When isolated	8	44	0	7	0	5	0	15	15	84	4	20	0	20	20	2	0	0	0
Miscellaneous	When isolated	34	41	3	17	0	4	0	4	17	20	0	15	7	7	7	0	0	0	6
"Lab." strains	Before and after animal passage	5	100	2	18	5	2	2	2	45	49	0	15	12	19	17	2	0	6	0
Average percentage of animals injected with non-specific strains showing lesions in individual organs				5	20	9	11	6	8	27	14	2	10	12	9	11	2	1	3	0

EXHIBIT B: PHOTOCOPY: HOLMAN'S 1928 "REARRANGEMENT"

Holman, W.L., Archives Path & Lab. Med. 5,133 (1928).

A Rearrangement of Rosenow's Results Showing Number of Animals with various Lesions and the Percentage of These Lesions Following the Injection of "Specific" and "Nonspecific" Strains of Streptococci

Number and Percentage of Animals Showing Various Lesions :	At Isola-tion	After Animal Later Passage		Totals
1. Lesions of the Joints				
Number of animals affected	131	28	37	196
Percentage with strains from patients with rheumatic fever	36	11	19	29
Percentage with other strains	64	89	81	71
2. Endocardial Lesions				
Number of animals affected	122	17	21	160
Percentage with strains from patients with endocarditis	30	..	..	23
Percentage with strains from patients with rheumatic fever	27	18	48	29
Percentage with other strains	42	82	52	48
3. Myocardial Lesions				
Number of animals affected	82	11	16	109
Percentage with strains from patients with rheumatic fever	38	36	44	39
Percentage with strains from patients with myositis	17	..	..	13
Percentage with other strains	44	64	56	48
4. Lesions of the Muscles				
Number of animals affected	78	13	19	110
Percentage with strains from patients with rheumatic fever	24	0	16	20
Percentage with strains from patients with myositis	38	..	..	27
Percentage with other strains	37	100	84	53
5. Stomach and Duodenal Lesions with Hemorrhages				
Number of animals affected	130	16	36	182
Percentage with strains from patients with ulcer of stomach	48	6	25	40
Percentage with other strains	52	94	75	60
6. Stomach and Duodenal Lesions with Ulcer				
Number of animals affected	92	10	27	129
Percentage with strains from patients with ulcer of stomach	67	0	48	58
Percentage with other strains	33	100	52	42
7. Lesions of the Gallbladder				
Number of animals affected	76	5	38	119
Percentage with strains from patients with cholecystitis	43	20	24	36
Percentage with other strains	57	80	76	64
8. Appendical Lesions				
Number of animals affected	65	8	14	87
Percentage with strains from patients with appendicitis	71	50	71	69
Percentage with other strains	29	50	29	31
9. Lesions of Kidneys				
Number of animals affected	54	5	16	75
Percentage with strains from patients with rheumatic fever	52	60	50	52
Percentage with other strains	48	40	50	48

Table 1a: ROSENOW RESULTS* v. HOLMAN "REARRANGEMENT"**

LESIONS from IN bacteria ANIMALS' \/ \/	SOURCE: PATIENTS WITH \/	Rosenow's Data ANIMALS INJECTED \/	% with lesions \/	(NO.W/LES.***)	Holman's Portrayal \/ \/
JOINTS					
as isolated					131
Rheumatic fever		71	66%	(= 47)	36%
***Other strains		437	19%	(= 84)	64%
later					28
Rheumatic fever		14	21%	(= 3)	11%
***Other strains		94	27%	(= 25)	89%
after animal passage					37
Rheumatic fever		19	37%	(= 7)	19%
***Other strains		98	31%	(= 30)	81%
total					196
Rheumatic fever		104	55%	(= 57)	29%
***Other strains		629	22%	(=139)	71%
ENDOCARDIUM					
as isolated					122
Endocarditis		44	84%	(= 37)	30%
Rheumatic fever		71	46%	(= 33)	27%
***Other strains		393	13%	(= 52)	42%
later					17
Endocarditis		–			–
Rheumatic fever		14	21%	(= 3)	18%
***Other strains		94	15%	(= 14)	82%
after animal passage					21
Endocarditis		–			–
Rheumatic fever		19	53%	(= 10)	48%
***Other strains		98	11%	(= 11)	52%
total					160
Endocarditis		44	84%	(= 37)	23%
Rheumatic fever		104	44%	(= 46)	29%
***Other strains		585	13%	(= 77)	48%
MYOCARDIUM					
as isolated					82
Rheumatic fever		71	45%	(= 32)	38%
Myositis		40	35%	(= 14)	17%
***Other strains		397	9%	(= 36)	44%
later					11
Rheumatic fever		14	29%	(= 4)	36%
Myositis		–			–
***Other strains		94	7%	(= 7)	64%
after animal passage					16
Rheumatic fever		19	37%	(= 7)	44%
Myositis		–			–
***Other strains		98	9%	(= 9)	56%
total					109
Rheumatic fever		104	41%	(= 43)	39%
Myositis		40	35%	(= 14)	13%
***Other strains		589	9%	(= 52)	48%

(continued)

Table 1a (continued)

LESIONS from IN bacteria ANIMALS' \/ \/	SOURCE: PATIENTS WITH \/	Rosenow's Data			Holman's Portrayal	
		ANIMALS INJECTED \/	% with lesions \/	(NO.W/LES.***)	\/	\/
MUSCLES						
as isolated					78	
	Rheumatic fever	71	27%	(= 19)		24%
	Myositis	40	75%	(= 30)		38%
	***Other strains	397	7%	(= 29)		37%
later					13	
	Rheumatic fever	14	0%			0%
	Myositis	—				—
	***Other strains	94	14%	(= 13)		100%
after animal passage					19	
	Rheumatic fever	19	16%	(= 3)		16%
	Myositis	—				—
	***Other strains	98	16%	(= 16)		84%
total					110	
	Rheumatic fever	104	21%	(= 22)		20%
	Myositis	40	75%	(= 30)		27%
	***Other strains	589	10%	(= 58)		53%
STOMACH/DUODENUM, WITH HEMORRHAGES						
as isolated					130	
	Stomach ulcer	103	60%	(= 62)		48%
	***Other strains	405	17%	(= 68)		52%
later					16	
	Stomach ulcer	22	5%	(= 1)		6%
	***Other strains	86	17%	(= 15)		94%
after animal passage					36	
	Stomach ulcer	39	23%	(= 9)		25%
	***Other strains	78	35%	(= 27)		75%
total					182	
	Stomach ulcer	164	45%	(= 73)		40%
	***Other strains	569	19%	(=109)		60%
STOMACH/DUODENUM, WITH ULCER						
as isolated					92	
	Stomach ulcer	103	60%	(= 62)		67%
	***Other strains	405	7%	(= 30)		33%
later					10	
	Stomach ulcer	22	0%			0%
	***Other strains	86	12%	(= 10)		100%
after animal passage					27	
	Stomach ulcer	39	33%	(= 13)		48%
	***Other strains	78	18%	(= 15)		52%
total					129	
	Stomach ulcer	164	46%	(= 75)		58%
	***Other strains	569	9%	(= 54)		42%
GALLBLADDER						
as isolated					76	
	Cholecystitis	41	80%	(= 33)		43%
	***Other strains	467	9%	(= 43)		57%
later					5	
	Cholecystitis	14	7%	(= 1)		20%
	***Other strains	94	4%	(= 4)		80%
after animal passage					38	
	Cholecystitis	16	56%	(= 9)		24%
	***Other strains	98	30%	(= 29)		76%

(continued)

Table 1a (continued)

LESIONS from IN bacteria ANIMALS' \/ \/	SOURCE: PATIENTS WITH \/	Rosenow's Data ANIMALS INJECTED \/	% with lesions \/	(NO.W/LES.***)	Holman's Portrayal \/ \/
total					119
	Cholecystitis	71	61%	(= 43)	36%
	***Other strains	662	11%	(= 76)	64%
APPENDIX					
as isolated					65
	Appendicitis	68	68%	(= 46)	71%
	***Other strains	440	4%	(= 19)	29%
later					8
	Appendicitis	26	15%	(= 4)	50%
	***Other strains	82	5%	(= 4)	50%
after animal passage					14
	Appendicitis	22	45%	(= 10)	71%
	***Other strains	95	4%	(= 4)	29%
total					87
	Appendicitis	116	52%	(= 60)	69%
	***Other strains	617	4%	(= 27)	31%
KIDNEY					
as isolated					54
	Rheumatic fever	71	39%	(= 28)	52%
	***Other strains	137	6%	(= 26)	48%
later					5
	Rheumatic fever	14	21%	(= 3)	60%
	***Other strains	94	2%	(= 2)	40%
after animal passage					16
	Rheumatic fever	19	42%	(= 8)	50%
	***Other strains	98	8%	(= 8)	50%
total					75
	Rheumatic fever	104	38%	(= 39)	52%
	***Other strains	629	6%	(= 36)	48%
SKIN as isolated					
	Erythema nodosum	20	90%	Not listed	
	Herpes zoster	61	70%	by Holman	
	***Other diseases	427	4%		
PAROTID					
as isolated					
	Mumps	19	73%	Not listed	
	***Other diseases	489	0%	by Holman	
PANCREAS					
as isolated					
	Mumps	19	42%	Not listed	
	***Other diseases	489	4%	by Holman	

*   Rosenow, E. C., J.A.M.A. LXV 1688 (1915).
**   Holman, W.L., Archives Path & Lab. Med. 5 (1928), 133.
*** Please note, as evident in Exhibit 1, that these totals were not provided in Rosenow's data, and each had to be laboriously calculated by Holman in order to proceed to his fraudulently deceptive presentation.

Table 2. ELECTIVE LOCALIZATION OF STREPTOCOCCI, 11,479 ANIMALS*

LESIONS IN ANIMALS'	SOURCE: DENTAL/OTHER FOCI IN PERSONS WITH	ROSENOW		ELEVEN CO-WORK.		TWENTY OTHERS		TOTALS	
		#	%	#	%	#	%	#	%
Stomach	Stomach/duodenum ulcer	1539	65	1231	52	280	60	3050	57**
	Other diseases	3341	8	1798	6	996	3	6135	06**
	No systemic disease	1329	14	665	7	300	7	2294	11**
Joints	Arthritis	1447	53	1225	58	415	59	3087	56
	Other diseases	3433	13	1804	7	861	39	6098	15
	No systemic disease	1329	18	665	11	300	31	2294	18
Eyes	Iritis, other eye dis.	272	42	328	43	186	53	786	45
	Other diseases	4608	1	2701	1	1090	1	8399	01
	No systemic disease	1329	8	665	0	300	2	2294	05
Myocardium	Myocarditis	36	61	39	38	94	59	169	54
	Other diseases	4844	3	2990	7	1182	11	9016	06
	No systemic disease	1329	6	665	3	300	17	2294	07
Muscles	Myositis	891	72	50	58	86	56	1027	70
	Other diseases	3989	6	2979	9	1190	12	8158	08
	No systemic disease	1329	3	665	7	300	13	2294	05
Kidneys	Pyelonephritis	168	73	96	83	96	58	360	72
	Other diseases	4712	6	2933	3	1180	16	8825	07
	No systemic disease	1329	9	665	7	300	19	2294	10
Colon	Ulcerative colitis	527	58	60	60	119	42	706	56
	Other diseases	4353	2	2969	0	1157	1	8479	01
	No systemic disease	1329	5	665	0	300	0	2294	03
	TOTALS	6209		3694		1576		11479	

* Rosenow, E. C., Dental Centenary Proceedings, Maryland State
   Dental Association and A.D.A., March 1940, p. 261-82.

** Example: In all 57% of 3050 animals injected with bacteria from patients with
stomach ulcers developed stomach ulcer lesions, vs. 6% of 6135 animals injected with
strains from other diseases, and 11% of 2294 animals injected with strains from
persons with no systemic disease.

<4> THE FALLOUT

CONTINUING IMPLICATIONS OF HOLMAN'S DECEPTION

Holman's 1928 article had been preceded by a letter to JAMA in 1927, wherein he first stated that the 1916 work of Rosenow "does not indicate more than a 50% chance for either specific or non-specific strains" to cause a given disease condition in laboratory animals." (See APPENDIX C for further details of Holman 1927) This assertion was repeated, and specific details claiming to support it were first provided, in Holman 1928. As revealed above in <2> "THE FACTS" and in Table 1, the statement is nothing but an incredibly audacious, weasel-worded deflection.

The pervasive historical and continuing impact of Holman's deception is illustrated in Figure 1: DEPTH OF DECEPTION. The works listed in Figure 1 are ALL so reliant (directly or indirectly) on the fraudulent presentation of Holman, as pertains to their rejection of Rosenow, so as to warrant their being purged from the literature; and rendering any works and/or practices which rely on them (as regards purported refutation of the value of the focal infection concept) to be also vitally flawed. For example, in Figure 1, "G" (Grossman, 1940) prominently cites items "A", "B", "C", and "D"; whereas "B" and "C" prominently cite "A" (Holman)"; and "D" cites both "A" and "B". It's a huge inverted pyramid perched atop a ludicrous fraud, a humongous iceberg the dimensions of which spreads far beyond the mere "B" through "Y" citations in Figure 1, one which occupies a significant sector of the mentality of modern dentistry, and by extension, a frighteningly large sector of modern medical theory and practice. In other words, it's time for a grand book burning.

So that the reader might gain an appreciation that this is indeed the case, Figure 1 is supported by a detailed compilation of excerpts/annotations from each of the items listed, as provided in APPENDIX C, "HOLMAN'S LEGACY - A CON CHRON". The tremendous scope of the continuing damning legacy of Holman's deception is particularly exemplified in item "R", Paul Beeson's (1976) authoritative American Bicentennial assessment, which characterized the focal infection works of Billings and Rosenow as *the* notable failure of American medicine this century; Beeson's influence on modern medical thought is further indicated by his designation, as per Science Magazine [Reines 1989], as the "doyen of American internal medicine". Yet the totality of Beeson's case against Rosenow rests firmly on Holman's Deception. Insofar as Beeson's position may be taken to epitomize the basis of conventional medical wisdom, so must this presumed "wisdom" be acknowledged to be severely tainted or even vitally flawed.

But this seemingly sad state of affairs is actually not cause for despair; rather, the revival of the monumental works of Billings and Rosenow, and their many other fine predecessors, associates and successors, is cause for great rejoicing. Yes, we do indeed have a firm grasp on the environmental-microbial, cause of MS, schizophrenia, arthritis, appendicitis, epilepsy, etc., etc., and

probably even AIDS. The broad and specific implications of these
works are discussed in greater detail in *REFERENCE MANUAL ROSENOW
ET AL.*

   As shown in Figure 1, Holman's grand deception continues to
support a humongous inverted pyramid of ignorance, with respect to
the established insidious nature of oral foci of infection
(diseased, including all nonvital, teeth and/or diseased tonsils),
within the essential foundations of modern medicine and dentistry.
 The individual items in Figure 1 are discussed in APPENDIX E - A
CON CHRON".

Figure 1: DEPTH OF DECEPTION

```
   Author ----      year   Key References Include:
A. Holman    1928
B. McNevin   1930   A
C. Blayney   1932   A
D. Appleton  1933   AB
E. Sharp     1937    B
F. Reimann   1940   A
G. Grossman  1940   ABCD
H. Woods     1942   A    FG
I. Grossman  1946   ABCD F H
J. Crowley   1946        FGH
K. Wolfson   1949    B       HI
L. Easlick   1951   A    FGHI
M. Jawetz    1955    B
N. Coolidge  1960     CD    I
O. Topazian  1962   A      G     L
P. Burket    1971   A    F   J LM
Q. Grossman  1976       G
R. Beeson    1976     F
S. Bellizi   1980           K
T. Chase     1980                    R
U. Ingle     1985                 Q
V. Grossman  1988     CD
W. Wiene     1989     CDE
X. Harty     1990   (Grossman positions paraphrased)
Y. Walton    1996   (No discussion of focal infection)
```

   A "VIRUS" LOOSE IN THE HISTORY OF MEDICINE

   A terrible "virus" is loose in the history of medicine and
dentistry -- in the literature and the retelling of the lessons of
history -- self-replicating and becoming more entrenched with every
new report, popular or professional, print or video or whatnot,
that, as a direct or indirect result of the Holman deception,
either degrades or ignores the Billings-Rosenow Syndrome and
Rosenow's proofs of elective localization of bacteria from oral
foci as a (the) key factor in the causation of a wide range of
diseases in genetically pre-disposed persons.

<5> EPILOGUE TO FRAUD - SHAME SHAME SHAME

It is difficult to understand how or why the whole gaggle of writers in Figure 1, DEPTH OF DECEPTION, particularly Beeson and most prominently Grossman, have managed to evade reference to Rosenow's four decades of substantiating work following his landmark (Holman-defrauded) 1915 article, and for ignoring and/or misrepresenting the wealth of prior and subsequent supporting publications by many others which had repeatedly validated Rosenow's work. Certainly the claim might be made that each was merely retelling "facts" as had been told by prominent predecessors. But these were not foot soldiers who would have been shot for not following orders. These are, or were, presumably the best and brightest among us, the best and brightest dentists and doctors. Yet, in their perpetuation of the Holman legacy, at a minimum through the simple failure to check their references and facts, they have contributed to the needless suffering and early death of thousands, even millions.

In fact the tremendous accomplishments of Billings and associates, including most prominently the truly monumental bacteriological works of Rosenow, have never been refuted and have much to offer in terms of augmenting and advancing current medical and dental knowledge. This particularly includes the etiologic importance of, and need to remove, infected teeth (including all, often-symptomless, pulpless teeth) and tonsils (particularly residually-infected previously-operated often-symptomless ones), and the advocacy of autogenous vaccine-therapy.

A key issue in much of the historical controversy over focal infection has concerned the pulpless tooth, pitting those who asserted that pulpless teeth could be sterilized and thus saved; against the assertions of Rosenow and others that sterility cannot be maintained in pulpless teeth and further that pulpless teeth (with or without symptoms) are often foci of particular etiologic importance. Regarding the present situation as concerns modern dentistry, contemporary endodontics (root-canal) textbooks continue to be heavily influenced by the Holman legacy (e.g., U, V, and W, above) as pertains to the question of etiological significance of symptomless pulpless teeth. To do otherwise would seem to fatally compromise the very profession of endodontics.

Of several contemporary endodontics textbooks reviewed as of 1996, only Cohen and Burns 1987, was found to incorporate some measure of balance into its presentation. Therein Morse states "... there are indications that secondary disease from an oral focus can occur." (Morse also relates "oral focus" to "autoimmune disease"; this is consistent with Rosenow's having long ago established that many diseases currently referred to as "autoimmune" are actually oral focal diseases.)

Also in Cohen and Burns 1987, Samuel Seltzer acknowledges that nonvital teeth are commonly infected, without further discussion as to how these may (and in fact do) comprise oral foci which cause systemic disease.

<6> NONVITAL TEETH ARE INFECTED

SUPPORTING ITEMS IN THE HISTORICAL RECORD:

  INFECTION IN FILLED, VITAL X-RAY NEGATIVE TEETH

   "Pulpless teeth, irrespective of whether they gave
roentgenographic evidence of changes, have proved to harbor
specific types of streptococci [which] on injection into animals,
tend to localize and produce disease resembling that of the
patient" [Rosenow 1944].
   The pathogenic role of symptomless, both roentgeno-graphically
positive and negative, pulpless teeth was repeatedly demonstrated
by E. C. Rosenow, and implicated in a number of disease conditions.

  IMPORTANCE OF SYMPTOMLESS FOCI

   "The causative streptococcus often was isolated not only from
badly infected tonsils but from tonsils that appeared small and
normal but which on removal were large and sometimes contained
abscesses, from unsuspected remnants of tonsils, and from
symptomless roentgenographically positive and negative pulpless
teeth, root tips and residual areas which had not been considered
previously or which were thought to be harmless." [Rosenow 1929]
- -
Table 3:   Foci of infection in:

Diseases:
                tonsils, teeth, pulpless teeth
encephalitis   70%   56%   87%
arthritis   51   69   61
torticollis   60   75   76
MS   78   67   89
chronic polio   65   71   92
gastroduod.ulcer 74   74   52
lesions of eye   53   53   50
lesions of skin   74   56   77
prostatitis   63   54   69

  THE INSOLUBLE PROBLEM OF APICAL ENDS

   Rosenow discussed at length the issue of non-vital teeth, with
specific mention of three supporting studies:
   (a) L.T. Austin and T.J. Cook, J.A.D.A. 16, May 1929, 894-6,
found that 89% of 100 pulpless teeth v. 4% of 100 vital teeth
yielded characteristic implicated streptococci.
   (b) P.S. Rhoads and G.F. Dick, J.A.D.A. 19, November 1932,
1884-93, reported that the number of colonies from the apexes of
pulpless teeth was 700 to 1000 times greater than the number
obtained from identically treated vital teeth; and
   (c) W.F. Swanson and L.E. Van Kirk, J. Dent. Research 15,
September 1936, p. 315, found that 96% of 1220 root-filled pulpless

teeth and 98% of 582 non-root-filled pulpless teeth yielded a
growth, chiefly green-producing streptococci. [Rosenow 1940]

Further details on Austin and Cook, Rhoads and Dick, and Swanson
and Van Kirk:
Austin and Cook 1929 sought "to secure a control for the large
number of pulpless teeth cultured at The Mayo Clinic, and to
determine the correctness of the opinion that a large percentage of
normal vital teeth yield cultures of streptococci". They used
normal vital teeth being removed because a full denture was being
advised, with no more than two teeth from any one case, using
extremely careful, described in detail, sterile methods. The vital
teeth were compared with identically-treated pulpless teeth, both
roentgenically negative and positive.

Table 4: Austin/Cook Comparison of Vital vs. Pulpless Teeth

Teeth	Number	Cultures G-B Broth %yes	%no	Cultures in Glucose-Brain Agar Zero Growth	Numbers of Colonies 0-20	20-50	50-100	100+
Vital	100	4	96	96	3	--	1	--
Pulpless	100	89	11	11	2	9	3	75
X-ray negative	50	84	16	16	4	8	2	70
X-ray positive	50	94	6	6	--	10	4	80

As seen in Table 4, above, most of the pulpless teeth, both x-ray
negative and positive, were shown to be generally infected, and
grossly so, when compared to the vital teeth.
Fully 96% of the vital teeth yielded no bacterial growth in
either of the two culture media. In three percent, minimal growth
was obtained, and in only one was moderate growth obtained.
"... A possible explanation for the 4 percent of positive
cultures [in vital teeth] may be that some of these cultures were
obtained from patients who were not only harboring a large number
of infected teeth, some of which were immediately adjacent to the
vital tooth cultured, but were also suffering from infective
diseases.
"In the pulpless group, which was used as a control, it was
interesting to note that there was not a great difference" between
x-ray negative and x-ray positive groups."
Of the pulpless teeth, not only did 89% yield a positive growth
of streptococci, but also "of this series, 75 per cent yielded more
than 100 colonies in agar, which indicated that considerable
infection was present in most of the cases."

PULPLESS TEETH - SUMMARIES OF 3000 PERSONS

Rhoads and Dick, 1932, undertook to study the pathologic
significance of pulpless roentgenographically negative teeth.
Summarizing studies involving more than 3000 persons, the authors
found "69.2% of pulpless teeth in adults had roentgenographic

evidence of periapical bone change. Assuming that root canal
filling is undertaken to preserve the teeth and conserve the
patient's health, these figures would indicated that the procedure
is unsuccessful in the hands of the majority of dentists."

ALL PULPLESS TEETH ARE PROBABLE FOCI

   Rhoads and Dick, 1932, cultured green-forming cocci from all of
209 roentgen ray negative pulpless teeth and concluded that "it
seems justifiable to regard all pulpless teeth as probable foci of
infection, whether they show apical change in the roentgenograms or
not. Certainly that position should be taken in the presence of
systemic disease of a type usually associated with focal
infection."

PULPLESS TEETH - 1800 OBSERVED

   Swanson and Van Kirk, 1936, cultured 1800 extracted, pulpless
teeth in brain-heart-infusion medium and observed:
   "Positive cultures [pure cultures of non-hemolytic diplo-
streptococci] resulted from enough x-ray negative [root-filled
pulpless] teeth to warrant the statement that absence of x-ray
evidence does not guarantee sterility in pulpless teeth. The small
difference in incidence of infection [96.4% for root-filled v.
97.8% for not-root filled] would seem to indicate, conversely, that
the sterile pulpless tooth under any circumstances may be an
extreme rarity." This referred to the authors having obtained
positive cultures in 96.4% of 1220 root-filled teeth and 97.8% of
582 not-root-filled teeth for an overall 96.8% of 1802 pulpless
teeth.
   The authors also extracted several pulpless teeth from a 77 year-
old encephalitis patient, cultured gram-positive streptococci which
were injected intravenously into a rabbit resulting in "definite"
disturbance of the central nervous system. This was repeated
through 6 animal passages, wherein affinity for the central nervous
system was retained.

MODERN CONFIRMATION, SO CHANGE THE SUBJECT?

   Seltzer 1987 [in Cohen and Burns] cites Blayney, Grossman and
others as having an impact on saving teeth, but concedes that in
the early 1970s "more sophisticated techniques, such as those using
strictly anaerobic conditions, revealed the presence of microorganisms that hitherto had been unreported in root canals. ...
numerous medicaments were advocated for killing the inhabitants of
the root canal. ... Obtaining subsequent negative cultures was
important evidence ... that endodontic therapy was capable of
sterilizing the root canal. ...
   "Unfortunately, it soon became apparent that negative cultures

did not necessarily reflect the true status of the root canal. Some culture reversals were detected. The emphasis on obtaining negative cultures began to be dissipated. In addition, because of culturing and other factors, treatment was time consuming. ...

"In the 1960s and 1970s, serious questions were raised about the necessity of obtaining negative cultures. [Note that Rosenow had died in 1966.] The emphasis began to shift from microbiology to the emerging field of immunology."

In other words, Seltzer acknowledges that non-vital teeth cannot be kept sterile - exactly what Rosenow and numerous independent and associated studies had maintained all along. The apparent response of endodontics has been to allow this previously all-important "emphasis" to "be dissipated", i.e., to ignore it and change the subject to "the emerging field of immunology". This simply ignores the fact that bacteria emanating through the bloodstream from these oral foci cause a wide range of systemic diseases, which is why endodontics from inception has necessarily insisted that non-vital teeth *could* be kept sterile. The fact is, as must be repeatedly and redundantly emphasized, they *cannot*.

The importance of sterility in non-vital teeth was not lost on even Louis Grossman, who notably continued to emphasize the importance of culturing them before filling to assure their sterility (e.g., see Grossman 1938, 1960 in APPENDIX F).

Once more, with emphasis: The fact is that there is now way to keep non-vital teeth sterile. Teeth which have undergone root-canal "therapy" are infected and will always be infected. They will always be a focus of infection in the person in whose mouth they remain, until they are removed or until the person dies. And they will likely, if not invariably, contribute to the hastening of the demise of the patients (victims) involved.

Practitioners of root-canal therapy are confronted with a clear and vital conflict of interest between the realization that pulpless teeth cannot be kept sterile and the (intrinsically flawed) commitment to saving pulpless teeth. However, until the "emerging field of immunology" is able to keep those organisms that grow at the base of non-vital or otherwise diseased teeth from continually entering the bloodstream and causing a wide range of chronic diseases, as has been clearly demonstrated by Rosenow and others (e.g., Haden 1928, Price 1923, Wilkie 1928, Nickel and Hufford 1928, etc., Seltzer would do well to advise his colleagues (1) against the ill-advised, deeply ingrained, teachings of their profession, to PULL ALL NON-VITAL TEETH, (2) to do so in a properly thorough manner, so as to remove residual jawbone infection and avert further jawbone degeneration (e.g., "cavitations"), (3) utilize Rosenow's methods of cultivation of properly-specific organisms and application of autogenous vaccine-therapy, prior and subsequent to removal of these foci, and (4) to immediately promote the use of bi-weekly (intramuscular) autohemotherapy by affected patients so as to minimize damage until more definitive solutions are effected, i.e., removal of primary (oral) foci and neutralization of secondary foci through specific (autogenous) vaccine-therapy.

ROOT-CANAL-TREATMENT PIONEER CLAIMS COVER-UP

   Beyond and without reference to Holman's fraud, George Meinig, D.D.S., a founding member of the American Association of Endodontists (root-canal-therapists), has alleged that opponents of the concept of focal infection suppressed facts concerning the role of devitalized teeth in systemic disease. (*Root Canal Cover-up*, Bion Publishing, P.O. Box 10, Ojai, CA 93024; www.meinig.com)
   Meinig has intensively reviewed the work of Weston Price (which essentially condemned root-canal "therapy"), and justifiably objects to not having learned of Price's and associated works during his education and subsequent long professional career as a dentist. According to Meinig, the "cover-up" seems to have been more subtle than overt.
   To some extent, pre-determined and well-ingrained professional attitudes may preclude fair consideration of the focal infection concept, with the same net result as a "cover-up". For example, in a 1994 review of focal infection, RA Hughes stated "attempts to repeat the isolation [and elective localization] work of Rosenow often failed to confirm his findings". Further down in the Hughes article, and without reference back, the author related that Rosenow's requisite "stringent, specific culture conditions ... were rarely observed by later investigators". Left unstated was the fact that when these conditions were met, Rosenow's work was invariably substantiated.
   Nor does there seem to be evidence of an actual overt conspiracy among pioneer root-canal-therapy advocates. Even in the case of Lewis Grossman, who certainly must be credited with having played a major role in the advocacy of root-canal therapy over the years, one would be inclined to assume he was motivated in the first instance by a desire to benefit patients through the advantage of retaining their own teeth.

GROSSMAN'S SUSTAINED PATTERN OF DECEPTION

   Yet, however honorable may have been Grossman's end purpose, actual scientific evidence supporting his position was lacking - so he essentially faked it. For example, from 1940 through 1988 his textbooks referred prominently to the well-respected bacteriological work of Haden 1928, without once mentioning the facts that: Haden's work was an exhaustive replication and validation of Rosenow's (as emphasized by former AMA President W. Bierring in *JAMA* 1938); and Haden had concluded that virtually all pulpless teeth should be extracted. (See also APPENDIX C: Grossman 1946, 1960, 1976, 1981, 1988; and supplementary items, APPENDIX E.)

   Even worse, in a special Jan. 1982 tribute issue of the *Journal of Endodontics*, Grossman's discussion of the founding of the American Association of Endodontists refers to "certain events" that allowed for the birth of the root-canal-treatment organization, citing two (and only two) articles: a June 1938 *JADA* editorial by C.N. Johnson, which Grossman refers to as a "turning point"; and a May 1940 *JADA* article by L.T. Austin of the Mayo Clinic, which Grossman sought to characterize as indicating a turn-around at Mayo on the question.

In essence, the Johnson editorial advised readers to simply ignore opposition (by "certain members of the medical profession") to root-canal treatment, in that "dentists had been studying the teeth for nearly a century ..."; the Austin article, from which Grossman excerpted reference to one (heart) investigator's reserved comments, was primarily comprised of overwhelming endorsements of the focal infection concept by several Mayo experts in various fields, including gastro-enterology, lower digestive tract, ophthalmology and genito-urinary tract. (In an earlier 1929 study , this same L.T. Austin had found that 89% of 100 pulpless teeth v. 4% of 100 vital teeth were infected with characteristic "focal infection"-associated disease-causing organisms).

These items are discussed in greater detail in APPENDIX F, "THE GROSSMAN FILE".

Yes, these two articles - the Johnson *JADA* editorial saying ignore the opposition, and the Austin article which actually indicts all pulpless teeth as relates to systemic disease - are the sum total of "certain events" offered up by Grossman as having set the stage for the birth of endodontics. In other words, it's a total sham, a hoax built on a fraud - a big, expensive joke.

The bottom line: At 20+ million "root-canals" a year, plus associated dental and medical bills down the road, till the road ends, this is a really big and expensive joke - a multi-billion dollar joke. (Estimate of 20+ million is based on: projection from data in *Survey of Dental Services Rendered*, ADA 1996, indicating root canal procedures by private practitioners increased from 6,790,000 in 1979 to 13,870,000 in 1990; and George Meinig, D.D.S., in *Root Canal Cover-Up*, who estimated more than 24 million root canals were treated in 1994. The figure may even be much larger; according to information put out by a private endodontics-clinic sponsor, the number may be up to 44 million per year, going up to 60 million by the year 2007.)

APPENDIX A: DISEASES DISCUSSED BY ROSENOW

Alcoholism
Alkaline phosphatic
  cystitis
Allergies
Amyotrophic lateral
  sclerosis
Anemia
Angina
Appendicitis
Arthritis
Asthma
Brain tumor
Bronchiectasis
Bronchitis
Bronchopneumonia
Cancer
Cholecystitis
Chorea
Colitis
Common Cold
Compulsive
  violence
Convulsions
Coronary heart
  disease
Cystic ovaries   Cystitis
Dermatology
Diabetes
Duodenal ulcer
Embolism
Encephalitis
Encephalomyelitis
Endocarditis
Endocervitis
Epilepsy
Erythema
Ether convulsions
Eye Diseases, e.g.,
  chorioretinitis
  glaucoma
  iridocyclitis
  iritis
  uveitis
Fibrositis
Gallbladder disease
Gallstones
Gastroenteritis
Gastric ulcer
Gastroduodenal
  ulcer

Goiter
Habit spasm
Hayfever
Headache (migraine)
Herpes
  Duhring's dis.
  simplex
  zoster
Hiccup, epidemic
  & post-operative
Hodgkins disease
Hyperpnea
  w/arrhythmia
Hypertension
Hypotension
Infertility
Influenza
Intercostal
  Neuralgia
Lethargy
Leukemia
Lobar pneumonia
Lupus erythematosus
Meningitis
Mental Illness
Mernier's disease
Migraine
Mononucleosis
Multiple neuritis
Multiple sclerosis
Mumps
Muscular dystrophy/
  atrophy
Myasthenia gravis
Myocardial lesions
Myoclonic
  encephalitis
Myositis
Nephritis
Nephrolithiasis
Nervous system
  diseases
Neuritis
Neuralgia
Neurofibromyositis
Neuromyositis
Osteitis deformans
Ovaritis
Paget's disease
Pancreatic disease

Parkinsonian
  encephalitis
Parotitis
Pemphigus
Periodic Ophthalmia
Pernicious anemia
Pneumonia
Pneumococcus
  infection
Poliomyelitis
Portal thrombosis
Prostatitis
Puerperal infection
Pulmonary diseases
Pulpitis
Pyelonephritis
Pyemia
Respiratory infect.
Rheumatic fever
Rheumatism
Scarlatinal
Scarlet fever
Schizophrenia
Sciatica
Sclerosis
Skin diseases
Sneeze, persistent
Sore throat
Spasmodic
Spasms during
  anesthesia
Splenic anemia
Stomach ulcer
Sydenham's Chorea,
  St. Vitus' dance
Thrombosis
Thyroiditis
  (exophthalmic)
Tonsillitis
Torticollis
Transverse myelitis
Trigeminal
  neuralgia
Ulcerative colitis
Ulcer
Urinary calculus,
  stone, tumor
Uveitis
Vagotonic neurosis
Venous thrombosis

Violent criminality
Zoster, Herpes
APPENDIX B: SOME ROSENOW TESTIMONIALS:

"Rosenow ... demonstrated in his laboratory an experiment on a single rabbit which was infected with material from a patient who had died under violent encephalitic hiccoughs. Already 48 hours after the injection, the animal died in front of the visitors eyes after having hiccoughed violently for several hours."
    [Jarlov E., Brinch O, Danish Section, *Assoc.Internationale Pour les Recherches sur la Paradentose, Copenhagen: Lassen and Stiedl*, 1938; abstr.- JAMA 111 (July 11, 1938), 290]

"Illingworth ..., using Rosenow's special medium, [showed that] streptococci could be grown from the wall of the gall bladder in quite a large percentage of cases in which the bile was sterile.
...
"... Dr. A. L. Wilkie ... has shown that cholecystitis is almost invariably an intramural streptococcal infection, and that Rosenow's contention of a selective affinity of this organism for the gall bladder is strikingly true. ... He has brought to light the illuminating and remarkable fact that bile inhibits the growth of this streptococcus. ... This fact accounts for the widespread failure to confirm Rosenow's findings. ...
    [Wilkie DPD, *Brit. Med. J.* 1 (1928), 481-4]

"Frick [A. Frick, *JAMA* 82:595 (Feb. 23, 1924] stated that according to his clinical experience there seems to be no doubt that Rosenow's theory of the elective affinity of a specific streptococcus ... for the gastric or duodenal mucosa is correct and that a specific streptococcus is the common cause of peptic ulcer."
"Eusterman [Eusterman GB, *Minn. Med.*, 6:698 (1923)] summarized the clinical evidence for the infectious origin of peptic ulcer in the light of recent experimental work and expressed the opinion that in certain types of ulcer it is the only tenable theory at this stage of medical progress." ...
"The streptococcus which we have isolated consistently in these cases is identical with that first described by Rosenow as having etiologic importance in the production of peptic ulcer in man, and it provides a means for active immunization with specific autogenous vaccine."
    [Nickel AC and AR Hufford, *Arch. Int. Med.* 41 (1928), 215.]

"Rosenow has shown us the various gradations of variety and morphology that different oxygen-pressures bring about, and has caught and held for our inspection the missing links of the chain of relationships between both acute and chronic bacillary and coccogenous affections."
    C. H. Pierce, *Journal-Lancet*, Minn., Aug. 1915, 414-9.

"It has long been known that the tendency of organisms to localize depends to a certain extent on virulence, and that the virulence of

an organism is changed by environment. Rosenow's elaboration has been so extensive, however, as to almost revolutionize former views concerning infection."
     William W. Duke, *Oral Sepsis in its Relationship to Systemic Disease*, Mosby, St. Louis, Mo. USA, 1918, 74.

"[Rosenow's] work has been so scientific, and his facts so firmly established that I believe we must either repudiate his facts, or in a general way accept his conclusion ... in regard to the elective affinity of bacteria for different organs and structures."
     George W. McCaskey in A.R. Barnes and A.S. Giordano, *Journal of Indiana State Med. Assoc.*, Ja. 15, 1922, 5.

"Rosenow made a fundamental contribution to bacteriology in demonstrating that the bacteria concerned in chronic foci of infection are very sensitive to oxygen tension, ... that the cultivation of the organisms and the reproduction of lesions in animals is largely dependent upon the use of proper laboratory technique [and] organisms in chronic foci vary greatly in their affinity for different tissues ... ."
     Russell L. Haden, *Dental Infection and Systemic Disease*, Lea and Febiger, Phila., Pa., 1928, 159.

"the tenets of both [bacteriology and immunology] offer definite confirmation [of specific tissue affinity], and perchance it is safe to assume that the 'Rosenow heresy' may yet become the medical guide of the future."
     Walter L. Bierring, 87th President of the A.M.A. (1934), in the *J.A.M.A.* 111 (Oct. 29, 1938), 1626.

 "[Rosenow] was adept at securing organisms from focal lesions, culturing them, and in reproducing the clinical syndromes of the patients in animals ... - especially tics of one kind or another. When the patient and the rabbit were placed side by side the resemblance of syndromes [was] often unbelievable and at times almost ludicrous and suggestive of plagiarism. ... he prepared autogenous vaccines that worked miracles in innumerable patients."
     Leonard G. Rowntree, *Amid Masters of Twentieth Century Medicine*, Charles C. Thomas, Springfield Ill. 1958

APPENDIX C: STANDARD OBJECTIONS AND REBUTTALS

A. REIMANN AND HAVENS 1940
B. HUGHES 1994
C. GROSSMAN'S KEY DIVERSIONS

A. REIMANN AND HAVENS 1940 ON INFECTED TEETH AND TONSILS

Because of its pivotal position in the literature, particularly vis-a-vis Beeson's 1976 Bi-Centennial bashing of the legacy of Billings and Rosenow, et. al., Reimann and Havens's 1940 "critical appraisal" of the focal infection concept seems to warrant particular scrutiny. Interestingly, in that same year, Martin Fischer [*Death and Dentistry*] had dismissed the Reimann and Havens article as a prime example of stupidity in its manner of rejection of Billings and his legacy.
   Nonetheless, Beeson's subsequent elevation of Reimann and Havens to the level of gospel has prompted the following a point-by-point examination of their 1940 "critical" appraisal, juxtaposed against Rosenow's 1940 presentation at the Dental Centennial, on some specific points of criticism raised by the former.

Infected Teeth, apical abscesses about ...

a. Bacteriologic studies

Reimann and Havens declared most studies of infection of pulpless teeth roots are invalid because of possible contamination.

   Rosenow 1940: "Slight contamination of teeth may occur during extraction, despite every precaution ...' [however] the much higher incidence of isolations from pulpless than from vital teeth simply cannot be referable to the aforementioned source of contamination."
   Here Rosenow refers to (p. 263) results of studies wherein 81% of 1382 pulpless teeth, when cultured in primarily dextrose-brain broth, were found to be infected by streptococci having elective localizing power, v. 38% of 548 vital teeth with no fillings or periodontoclasia.
   [Notably, Reimann and Havens, p. 2, cite a confirming study wherein, after tooth extraction, S. viridans was recovered in 75% of cases with obviously infected mouths v. 35% of apparently healthy mouths."]

b. Roentgenologic studies

Reimann and Havens 1940 assert that: Abnormal areas of lucency around the roots of teeth may not be caused by infection, but may nonetheless result in the loss of sound teeth.

   Rosenow 1940 concurred that: "Roentgenographically positive are usually, but not always, infected teeth. ... However, ... roentgenographically negative teeth are still nearly always considered sterile and harmless and are allowed to remain, despite the fact that they have been shown by methods to be infected by streptococci having elective localizing power in most instances in which patients are suffering from mild or severe systemic disease. ...

"Streptococci isolated from roentgenographically negative pulpless teeth in my experience have been more specifically virulent than those isolated from roentgenographically positive teeth. ... Improvement, often permanent, following removal of foci from which the causative streptococci were isolated in my experiences, have occurred with such regularity that I have come to consider lack of improvement as evidence that the removal was faulty, that the focus did not contain the causative micro-organism or that other foci were overlooked." (White in 1928 had made a similar observation in the case of optic neuritis and other diseases of the eye, having expressed disappointment when an oral focus was not immediately evident.)

c. Inoculation experiments

Reimann and Havens refer to Holman's 1928 review of elective localization as having concluded that the specificity of bacteria has not been proved, p. 1:

"Inoculation experiments - Most of the observations made on animals inoculated with bacteria recorded in studies of focal infection were reviewed by Holman in 1928. He particularly dealt with the problem of elective localization of bacteria and concluded that the specificity of the bacteria involved has not been proved and that the theory of Rosenow is open to misinterpretation and limited in its practical application."

Notably no reference was made to the fact that the point with which Holman "particularly dealt" involved a blatantly fraudulent statistical "rearrangement" at its heart, nor to Rosenow's numerous subsequent articles which voluminously and unequivocally addressed any and all substantive challenges to his work (Rosenow published an additional 73 articles between 1929 and 1939 inclusive, to which Reimann and Havens made absolutely no reference).

Rosenow 1940, p. 269, exhibits results of studies by himself, eleven co-workers and 22 other investigators involving over 11,000 animals, and which conclusively demonstrate the validity of the concept of elective localization as expounded by Rosenow.

d. Effect of extraction on systemic disease

Reimann and Havens 1940 note the existence of "... reports of clinical improvement after the extraction of a tooth .... Many such recoveries are temporary and may result from psychic factors or the shock-like reaction which often follows such operations. No one doubts that prompt improvement occasionally occurs after the extraction of suspected teeth. ... Many ophthalmologists ... feel that about 1/3 cases of iritis are due to focal infection, yet little or no proof exists for this belief, except the improvement which occasionally follows the extraction of teeth." The authors cite dangers of tooth extraction.

Rosenow 1940, p. 263, "The lack of striking clinical effects from elimination of focal infection is often attributable to the fact that even now the attempts are too often made after the disease process has continued for a long time and secondary foci such as in and about arthritis joints have become thoroughly established."
p. 264, Rosenow emphasized, relative to such diseases as cardiac disease, "how far from accurate purely clinical observations may be concerning the etiologic importance of symptomless foci, especially pulpless teeth which are normal in the roentgenogram, most of them with fillings in the canals of the roots." Rosenow asserts that exacerbations incident to extraction constitute proof that the theory is correct, i.e., that these bacteria are causative.

The Tonsils

a. "Infected tonsils"/tonsillectomy

Reimann and Havens, 1940, on tonsils, p. 4-5: "Tonsillectomy, like extraction of teeth, may lead to temporary bacteriemias, or in certain cases to subacute bacterial endocarditis. ... Numbers of cases of poliomyelitis have developed shortly after tonsillectomy. Numerous other conditions, diseases and relapses may be precipitated by tonsillectomy. ... It is generally admitted that occasional improvement does occur after operation on supposed infected areas, and many physicians are able to recite their own experiences of prompt relief of this or that complaint after the extraction of a tooth or after tonsillectomy. Such examples suggest, but by no means prove, an etiologic relationship. ...

Rosenow 1940 points out that such exacerbations further support the concept of focal infection, as discussed by Rosenow. Further, the connection between "numerous other conditions, diseases", etc., is further supportive of the Rosenow position.

b. Tonsillitis and Rheumatic Fever

On the question of acute rheumatic fever, Reimann and Havens indicate support of the concept that it is caused by tonsillitis: "... Davis does not believe that the tonsils are significant foci of infection for this disease. If they were, he believes, the number of tonsillectomies performed during the past 20 years should have reduced the incidence of rheumatic fever by now. It must be said however, that other studies have shown a diminished incidence of the disease, but the cause for it is not clear." Regarding rheumatic fever in children, the authors refer to Kaiser as having cited a "slight apparent advantage (2%) possessed by tonsillectomized children."
"The frequency with which acute rheumatic fever is preceded by an

attack of acute hemolytic streptococcus tonsillitis suggests to many an etiologic relationship of the bacteria to rheumatic fever."

B. HUGHES 1994:

Hughes 1994 conceded that "scientifically sound research ... [was] performed by a small number of highly motivated bacteriologists", this being the work from 1904 by Frank Billings and associates, particularly E.C. Rosenow, and Charles Mayo. Hughes relates a remarkable story told by Ejnar Jarlov, a previously skeptical Danish rheumatologist, of how Rosenow had replicated symptoms of an expired patient's violent hiccough in a rabbit.

However, Hughes' presentation overall is nonetheless somewhat negatively prejudicial and misrepresentative. For example, it:
(1) classes "focal infection" therapy as having been proved "ineffective" and "aimed at eradicating occult septic foci from the body"
WHEREAS these statements are simply false; no supporting documentation is given, undoubtedly because it does not exist.
(2) provides no Rosenow citations after 1923; refers to "later" research by others in 1928; and places a 1949 article as after "Rosenow's time".
WHEREAS this completely misrepresents the fact that Rosenow continued constructively working and publishing through 1958, and totally ignores his compilation of an irrefutable body of work.

Hughes specifically lists three major categories of "unanswered questions" and states these had led to skepticism over the concept of focal infection:

(1) "the true benefits of the removal of focal infection were never proven in suitable studies"
WHEREAS, Hughes himself refutes his statement, citing a 1922 Billings statistical report wherein removal of foci in arthritic patients had resulted in improvement in 69% of patients treated. Moreover as early as 1912 Billings had noted "The result of the removal of these infections has been most astounding in many instances." No mention is made of other confirming subsequent work, particularly that of Rosenow over the following 35 years, nor of Rosenow's repeated admonition that insofar as secondary foci may have become well established, a cure should not be expected in the case of removal of a primary focus of long-standing. [e.g., see Rosenow 1934]
(2) "the true incidence of focal sepsis in patients with inflammatory arthritis was never compared with that of normal controls during Rosenow's time", implying that Rosenow's work was deficient.
WHEREAS, much of Rosenow's work, as appropriate, involved comparisons with normal controls. In and of itself Rosenow's three-decades'-tenure with the Mayo Foundation is forceful

testimony against such attempts to imply that Rosenow's procedures were faulty. (e.g., see *REFERENCE MANUAL ROSENOW ET AL*)
     (3) "attempts to repeat the isolation [and elective localization] work of Rosenow often failed to confirm his findings"; however, Hughes does concede that the requisite *"stringent, specific culture conditions ... were rarely observed by later investigators."*

WHEREAS, when these conditions were met, Rosenow's work was invariably substantiated, including his demonstrations of the elective localization of streptococci. The bottom line on the subject is that these later investigators were/are either just too lazy or not interested in the facts; Hughes in trying to soft-pedal this and pejoratively come down on the anti-Rosenow side is, while seemingly reserving a professional courtesy-benefit-of-doubt for the anti-Rosenow charlatans, nonetheless behaving in a manner supportive of allegations of cover-up.

C.   GROSSMAN'S KEY DIVERSIONS
       (1) RED HERRINGS AND ANIMAL EXPERIMENTS
       (2) WEAK CONTAMINATION ARGUMENT IS KEY TOOL

(1) RED HERRINGS AND ANIMAL EXPERIMENTS

   GROSSMAN ARROGANTLY RIDICULES ROSENOW Grossman 1976
   After briefly discussing the early work of Hunter of England in the early 20th century, which increased awareness of the general role of oral infections, Grossman offered:
   "To add fuel to the fire, reports from bacteriologic laboratories began to come in that purported to show that infected teeth were a menace to health - the health of laboratory animals. It was an emotional period and no cognizance was taken of the fact that the amount of broth cultures injected into the animal was so large that it was no wonder the animal's health was overwhelmed. ... "

   RED HERRING! The fact is that the bacteria did electively locate in respective tissues of animals corresponding to diseased tissues of human host; moreover as early as 1919 and 1921 Rosenow had published studies using smaller doses specifically in response to critics of earlier large doses:
       - Rosenow, E.C., Focal infection and elective localization of
         bacteria in appendicitis, ulcer of the stomach, cholecystitis,
         and pancreatitis. Surg., Gynec., and Obst. 33:19-26, 1921:
         "My original experimental studies in ulcer, cholecystitis,
         and appendicitis extended over a short period, and included a
         relatively small series of cases. ... The number of bacteria
         injected was relatively large and this has been objected to.
         I believed it worthwhile, therefore, to continue the studies
         in a larger and more varied series, including recurrent ulcer,
         and to study the effect of the injection of smaller doses of
         bacteria. ... In all cases the symptoms were active at the
         time of the study and in all there were foci in which a
         [causal] relationship was suspected. Painstaking effort was

made to obtain cultures from the depths of the focus and to eliminate as far as possible the more saphrophytic bacteria on the surface. Glucose-brain broth in tall columns was substituted for ascites-glucose broth. The dose for a routine injection consisted of from 0.1 cc to 0.25 cc for each 100 grams of body weight. Usually only one injection was given. In order to rule out all possible objections to dosage, the small amount of pus expressed from tonsils and emulsions of tonsils was injected directly.

In this study, involving 183 strains of bacteria and 774 laboratory animals, bacteria from predominantly oral foci of persons with various diseases, including stomach ulcers, cholecystitis, appendicitis and myositis, were found to overwhelmingly electively locate in lab-animals' tissues which corresponded to the human systemic diseases.

See also - Rosenow, E.C., Studies on elective localization. Focal infection with special reference to oral sepsis. Jour. Dental Res. 1:205-267, 1919.

(2) WEAK CONTAMINATION ARGUMENT IS KEY TOOL

According to Grossman 1981:
"One of the most important researches dealing with bone infection which has a direct bearing on the treatment of pulpless teeth was contributed by Fish and MacLean of England."

Grossman states, on p. 140, that Fish and MacLean destroyed the microorganisms in the gingival sulcus (pocket) "by cauterizing the gingival tissue around the tooth to be extracted with a red hot cautery wire. ... Upon incubation, no growth of organisms was observed in the cultures from root apices [two incisors total], and the blood cultures were also sterile. ... In this manner it was established that apical tissues around the root of a periodontally involved tooth, though inflamed, were sterile and that organisms cultured from the root apices of such teeth or from the bloodstream after extraction had been pumped into the vessels of the periodontal ligament from the pocket during the preliminary loosening of the tooth in an effort to dislodge it from its alveolus. In a sense their work has negated all the bacteriologic studies of both pulpless and vital teeth when cultures were taken from the root surfaces or from tooth sockets following extraction."

Grossman, p. 146, repeats his claim, made since 1940 that "The work of Okell and Elliot and that of Fish explains the frequent isolation of microorganisms from both vital and pulpless extracted teeth. [Note that neither study involved pulpless teeth!] Their work negates all bacteriologic studies reported prior to 1936 since the gingival tissue was not cauterized in such studies in order to destroy the microorganisms in the gingival sulcus just prior to tooth extraction."

In other words, over an incredible half-century of arrogant ignoration of contrary facts, Grossman (from 1940-1988) attempts to enshrine as fact Fish and MacLean's lame speculation concerning possible contamination (based on the study of four teeth from one

patient, not involving gradients of oxygen pressure or other
requisite aspects of Rosenow's method, and not involving pulpless
teeth) and asserts that this is sufficient cause to throw out
everything else, including Rosenow's irreproachable career, his
nearly 300 articles over five-plus decades, and numerous confirming
works by others.

The type of argument advanced by Grossman, in his case an
inappropriate and frivolous subterfuge, may ironically be aptly
directed against his position and the overall question of root-
canal treatments. Insofar as the literature in favor of
endodontics is in fact dependent on Holman's fraud for its
scientific justification, the whole body of literature is in fact
mortally tainted and must be rejected, exposing root-canal
"therapy" (and with it much of modern dentistry) as what it is, the
most outrageous form of quackery ever foisted on humanity.

Grossman's two "key" referred articles on the subject of
contamination are discussed further below in APPENDIX D - THE
STERILITY ISSUE, along with some particularly relevant examples of
contrary evidence. Please bear in mind in reviewing these items
that Grossman et al. had sought to invalidate all contrary work via
reference to these two items (Okell and Elliot and Fish and
MacLean), including all of the works discussed above in <6> NON-
VITAL TEETH ARE INFECTED, and more - - everything contrary to the
Grossman position of endodontics advocacy.

APPENDIX D: THE STERILITY NON-ISSUE

A.   FOUNDATIONS OF THE GROSSMAN POSITION ON CONTAMINATION

- OKELL AND ELLIOT 1935
- FISH AND MACLEAN 1936

ADMITTEDLY "VERY INCOMPLETE" STUDY   Okell and Elliot 1935

Okell and Elliot 1935 seek to provide "a tentative explanation of how streptococci could reach the heart valves in cases of bacterial endocarditis", originating in oral foci and traveling through the bloodstream.

From the outset the authors state: "our object has been to confirm by direct observation ... what Lewis and Grant ... refer to as an 'almost physiological entry' of organisms into the blood stream of the average individual."

(We may note that insofar as all of the patients studied by Okell and Elliot required extractions, their results could not possibly reflect the physiology of "average" persons without oral foci.)

Okell and Elliot did not specifically refer to pulpless teeth, although they did observe that "in persons with severely septic mouths non-haemolytic streptococci may enter the blood stream in the absence of any obvious trauma. Owing to difficulties of access to patients our own observations on this point are very incomplete. We have been unable to ascertain whether the condition of 'leak' into the bloodstream in the positive cases is continuous, intermittent, or merely a fortuitous single occurrence."

Without reference to Rosenow's proofs of specific affinity by bacteria, Okell and Elliot conclude that the determining factor in bacterial endocarditis (acknowledged to be caused by bacteria from oral foci) is not the type of organism but rather "damage or malformation of the valves" (susceptibility). It may be noted that they do not appear to utilize the culture technique of Rosenow and thus were not working with the properly pathogenic organism demonstrated by Rosenow to have a specific affinity for heart valves in any case, nor did they attempt to do so.

It may be noted that Fischer 1940 [p. 228] refers to Okell and Elliott as having "noted a streptococus viridans bacteremia in sixty-one percent of 138 patients immediately after extraction with the 'amount of damage done' at operation held responsible for their highest counts." Fischer regards such bacteriemias to not contraindicate operations, but rather as argument that the patient be properly prepared, and that the physician use gentle surgical technic. The presumption, and fact, is that these extractions were necessitated by the existence of infected teeth, which would in most if not all circumstances be accompanied by a measure of infection in the surround jawbones; this explains the source of the resulting bacteriemias.

Overall, the use by Grossman of Okell and Elliot as evidence of contamination by Rosenow et. al. increasingly seems to be an argument bordering on the absurd.

FISHING FOR BACTERIA   Fish and MacLean, 1936

Fish and MacLean acknowledge the dangers of extraction, and the value of vaccine in mitigating it:
 "The healthy man with sciata may ... be allowed to run the inevitable but negligible risk of septicaemia from extraction, but if we have a patient with the same dental condition who is already delicate and ill and has perhaps nonvital, but as yet uninfected [wrong!], teeth [and] vegetations on the heart valve, it would be well to give her a course of vaccines before extracting the dead teeth or indeed before any surgical interference at all, so that she may the more readily kill any organism which is dislodged and prevent its settling on the damaged valves. ...
 "With apical infection we have at present no means of ensuring that the organisms shall not break loose into the bloodstream as the tooth gives way, and the danger to the patient can only be mitigated by prolonged artificial immunization with an autogenous vaccine."
 Fish and MacLean, 1936, p. 352-3, discuss the extraction of four teeth from the same patient, two cauterized and two not prior to extraction. No mention is made of the method of culture. Reference is made to supporting evidence based on other teeth examined post-mortem, but details are not provided. The authors purposefully excluded dead or pulpless teeth from their study:
 "Over two hundred extracted human teeth have been examined ... . There are also many dead or pulpless teeth. The dead teeth and those showing acute inflammation are not for the moment material to this inquiry, since it is known that streptococci are often pushed into the pulp mechanically through an exposure, and the result, as one would expect, is an acute abscess ... ."
 [In other words, their study was from the outset flawed by a pre-conceived incorrect hypothesis concerning infection in pulpless teeth, i.e., that found therein are the result of having been "pushed" in mechanically; further flawed by the small number of teeth examined; and independently refuted in a larger study by Tunnicliff and Hammond as discussed below. Fish and MacLean then asserted that results from their assessment of a few vital teeth "corroborate the interpretation we have placed on ... infected apices of dead teeth." The authors stated their opinion that "it seems to be a pathological impossibility to have streptococcal infection actually persisting in the bone lacunae and amongst the bone cells without necrosis. Similarly we cannot picture organisms living in the pulp without an acute or at least a chronic abscess; and yet we have the undoubted fact that the apices and the pulps of almost all teeth extracted in the ordinary way ... exhibit organisms bacteriologically which can be cultivated. The only explanation would appear to be that these organisms gain access to the tissues in some artificial way during extraction. This possibility was therefore investigated."
 Seemingly requiring clarification is their statement, p. 360, that "In the case of infected dead teeth the infection is confined

to the root canals or the pus of an associated chronic abscess. The surrounding bone and soft tissues are sterile though irritated by diffusible toxic products."

Something is wrong here. If an area is "irritated by diffusible toxic products", it is not sterile. Whereas using Rosenow's methods, these areas would be clearly demonstrated to be not sterile; the toxic products would be shown to yield S. rosenow, which could be further linked to systemic diseases of the respective patient; and so long as the blood supply is not cut off, which does not seem likely in any case until the patient dies, the infection "confined to" the root canals would and does in fact continually leak out into the blood stream and cause systemic disease.

B. MORE EVIDENCE OF THE FLAWED NATURE OF GROSSMAN'S POSITION

        - HENRICI AND HARTZELL 1919
        - TUNNICLIFF AND HAMMOND 1937
        - ROSENOW'S CAREFUL METHODOLOGY 1938

Henrici and Hartzell 1919, in a study involving (sterilely removed) pulps from "clinically vital teeth with grossly normal roots", comparing teeth with pyorrhea, caries or both, against "entirely normal" teeth, found infection in zero of 22 normal teeth, vs. 42% of 40 teeth with pyorrhea, 43% of 23 teeth with caries, and 46% of 30 teeth with both pyorrhea and caries.

"... in approximately one-half the number of vital teeth invaded by caries or surrounded by pyorrhea, the pulp is already infected by streptococci, a conclusion so startling that we felt some hesitancy about placing our work on record at this time. Nevertheless, we can find no fault in our technique, supported as it is by a series of twenty-two normal controls with uniformly negative results.

"The route of invasion of the pulp from caries is clearly along the dentinal tubules, and from pyorrhea it must be, as Collins and Lyne state, 'by extension from the gingival tissues.' We have referred in previous papers to lymphatic channels extending from the gingival region through the peridental membrane to the apical region. ..."

"From the results of our studies it would seem that the invasion and destruction of the pulp is frequently a long drawn out process, microorganisms being present long before actual necrosis of the tissues takes place. ..." [*J. Dent. Research* 1:419-422 (Dec.) 1919]

It is noted that Hartzell was a particularly prominent dentist in the early years of the Twentieth Century, and an active and well-regarded participant in the works of the early American Dental Association, serving as its president in 1922. This is highlighted both from the standpoint of the unchallengability of his work as in any way reflecting a contrarian position; and even moreso as an example of the fine work of many dentists within the A.D.A. throughout its history, and the proper motivation of most persons who have chosen to pursue careers in dentistry from the earliest times up to the present.

Tunnicliff and Hammond 1937 "examined pulps from thirty intact teeth the outside of which had been proved sterile", finding bacteria in ten, or 33%. They noted that there were "no signs at all of infection as indicated by leukocytic infiltration. When bacteria were present, they were generally in such large numbers as to suggest multiplication in the pulp during the eight days' incubation of the tooth. They were present generally in clumps in a circumscribed area ... "

The authors note that Fish and Maclean had asserted that bacteria found in extracted teeth had been pumped "by way of the periodontal membrane", and that prior cauterization would eliminate this. "Unfortunately, they cultured only three pulps. Although the pulps cultured by us were all from teeth extracted without cauterization, only 33 percent of the sterile teeth showed streptococci in the pulp."

The authors concluded that in these instances, "Since no sign of infection was observed in smears or sections of pulps containing streptococci, their presence is considered of no significance."

Without spelling it out in detail, the authors seem to have suggested that the bacteria may have been transient visitors in the bloodstream which happened to have been trapped within the involved teeth by the act of extraction. The commonsense presumption would be that these circumstances involved persons who had infected teeth or whatnot in the neighborhood, from which the transient hematogenous organisms had come. From this perspective, it seems particularly notable that fully two-thirds of the cases showed no growth of streptococci, given the likelihood of oral infection elsewhere in the mouths of the involved persons. [Tunnicliff, Ruth and Carolyn Hammond, "Presence of Bacteria in Pulps of Intact Teeth", *J.A.D.A. and Dental Cosmos* 24: 1663-1666 (Oct) 1937]

Regarding Rosenow's own work and the likelihood of contamination, the statement may be safely made that of all investigators Rosenow's was least subject to criticism on these grounds. The extreme precautions taken by Rosenow, seeking to avoid contamination, are exemplified in this excerpt from a 1938 article [Arch. Path. 26: 70-76, July 1938]: "Cultures were made under sterile conditions, either in a hood equipped with a glass shield and a copper roof, which radiates heat from the Bunsen burner, without change of air, and in which the air and the walls were sterilized with a fine spray of solution (1:1000) of mercuric chloride or a saturated solution of phenylmercuric chloride, or in a hot air sterilizer equipped with a glass shield and in which the air was sterilized by heat. All materials used in making the cultures and the mediums placed in the hoods were sterilized immediately before."

Contrast this with the "scientific" methods of Grossman, as for example discussed in his cute-puppy experiments in APPENDIX F - THE GROSSMAN FILE, and ... not much more need be said.

APPENDIX E: A CON CHRON - THE "CONS" OF FOCAL INFECTION

   In considering the historical record concerning merits of the
concept of focal infection (the "pros and cons", if you will), it
becomes clear that a distinct body of literature has emerged in the
current (20th) century in opposition. This curious phenomenon
seems to set off the "modern" era as probably the darkest of ages
in terms of recognition of the validity of this venerable concept.
   This section is comprised primarily of annotated excerpts from
this contrary body of literature, accessed in the course of
investigating Holman's 1928 fraudulent misrepresentation of
Rosenow's 1915 data. Not all of the comments are negative; on the
contrary, much of the following actually supports the concept of
focal infection, e.g., many of the items are mixed. In these
cases, the apparent only justification for fence sitting is
Holman's fraud. This seems particularly the case regarding Kolmer
1952 and a 1952 JAMA editorial, where just about everything about
the focal infection concept is considered valid, except Rosenow's
"theory" of elective localization. For that reason, although many
of these items have much positive to say on the concept, they are
included here in this "con" chron.
   This writer has searched and searched, and the reader is
cordially invited to join in the search, for anything beyond Holman
1927-1928 that supports rejection of Rosenow's exhaustive proofs of
the elective localization of organisms from oral foci as an
etiological factor in a wide range of diseases. Beyond Holman,
which is a total sham, it simply doesn't exist.
   And beyond Holman, one must review the work of L.I. Grossman.
As one gets further into it, Grossman's incredible and sustained
pattern of deception begins to make Holman's fraud seem trivial,
were the latter not so pivotally foundational for the remainder of
the literature. Brief references in this file are made to key
Grossman items in this historical series, i.e., particularly
Grossman 1940, 1946, 1976, 1981, and 1988; more detailed
discussions of these and the overall works of Grossman are
discussed in APPENDIX F: THE GROSSMAN FILE.
   But the problem did not begin with Holman, or Grossman. Even
earlier we find precedents for Grossman's single-minded advocacy in
the pre-Holman writings of future A.D.A. President Percy Howe in
1919 and by M.L. Rhein in 1926, both in the journal *Dental Cosmos*
(which Journal would be merged into *J.A.D.A.* in the 1930s), as
discussed below in the first items in this section.
   That the pejorative sentiments of Howe and Rhein were not
isolated opinions, but rather reflective of A.D.A. officialdom, is
forcefully exhibited in a subsequent section, APPENDIX G: JADA -
THE EARLY YEARS. Therein are highlighted the relevant works of
A.D.A. President J. P. Buckley, J.A.D.A.'s first editor Otto U.
King, and above all A.D.A. President and long-time J.A.D.A. editor
Charles N. Johnson. Thus it is clear that official dentistry was
fertile ground for Holman's deception of 1927-8.

HOWE CONCEDES FOCAL CONCEPT CONDEMNS DENTISTRY

Howe 1919 begins with the provocative overstatement that, if the "focal theory of infection ... is sound, ... [then] Wholesale extraction is demanded; an edentulous condition can be the only safe one, and dentistry stands condemned."

He commences to challenge the principle of focal infection based on the absence of arthritis deformans in school children with abscessed teeth. [But arthritis had been shown to be a chronic condition caused by long-standing oral infections, over periods of many years or decades, and thus would not be expected to be found in children.]

He then proceeds to emotional quips of "one distinguished man" who said "We still have 25 feet of intestines and five inches of mouth", not the reverse, and another who said "if teeth have much to do with disease the whole English race would have been exterminated long ago."

HOWE CHALLENGES SCIENCE WITH RHETORIC

He then refers derogatorily and incorrectly to "that group of bacteriologists who have made an especial study of the streptococcus" as having "selected the streptococcus viridans as the causative agent" [whereas in fact the streptococcus itself had done the selecting of tissues to eat and in which to cause disease, and the bacteriologists were there to observe it].

He then suggests that the bacteria that causes gastric ulcer is as likely to cause pyorrhea as the reverse, avoiding, or diverting attention from, Rosenow's demonstrations that organisms from oral foci cause specific diseases in animals which correspond to the human diseases of the hosts.

Howe later suggests that the specificity found in bacteria in oral foci is acquired in distant locations, and this specificity happens to be secondarily reflected in organisms taken from the oral foci. This, suggests Howe, is why bacteria from an extracted tooth in a Rosenow patient with appendicitis caused appendicitis in lab animals. [Indeed, specificity must develop as a result of communication between the oral and distant foci, whereby some of a range of organisms from the oral focus find a weak link in which to start a secondary colony, which then stimulates growth within the oral focus of these same strains. But without the focus, the disease would not have begun or proceeded.]

Howe also refers to one investigator's inability to replicate Rosenow's results with a streptococcus. Details are not given, not even the name of this investigator; however, we can assume that insofar as the numerous investigators who complied with Rosenow's procedures invariably obtained the same results, that incorrect procedures were used in the study referred to by Howe.

Howe challenges the significance of positive x-rays, those which seem to indicate infection, as not being alone sufficient to justify extraction of teeth. He concludes with "a protest against the indiscriminate extracting of teeth for their effect upon general diseases", which statement would find no greater supporter than Rosenow, who had steadfastly maintained that vital teeth without fillings or gum disease were invariably sterile and should be retained, and further that most but not all roentgenically positive teeth were infected.

It is particularly noted that the pulpless tooth is briefly mentioned on the first page of Howe's article, but not again. Hence, as this article was seemingly intended and has served as argument for the retention of pulpless teeth and in support of root-canal treatment and filling, it is unfortunately primarily not an exposition of arguments on that issue but rather is clearly an exercise in diversion.

DISEASED TEETH CAUSE DISEASE - OLD NEWS IN 1926 Rhein 1926

Rhein ML, et al., 1926, p. 970, "From our earliest available records, celebrated physicians in every era have written of diseased teeth as the cause at times of certain diseases. The fact that these empiric deductions were made in different centuries by physicians of so great renown that their names will forever be entwined in the history of medicine, is collaborating evidence of the soundness of their observations. ... It is a well established observation that a large proportion of these [dental focal] infections may exist for years without giving evidence of systemic disease, and then suddenly the previous good health of the patient is shattered,"

p. 972 "The fact should be borne in mind that the dental focal infections are usually of coccal origin, and the chief offending bacteria are most frequently S. viridans and other kinds of streptococci which grow on a blood culture with a green color and do not hemolyze the blood-culture medium. Now it happens that the body, on the whole, becomes poorly immunized to the cocci, a great deal more poorly indeed than to the bacilli. ... Hence ... the coccal infections arise over and over again in the same individual, as in furunculosis, sore throat, sinus infections, bronchitis, etc.

So also the dental focal infections, once started, are slow to subside, tend to persist, and ... often unexpectedly 'light up' and do much damage."

DIFFERENT CULTURE PROCEDURE, DIFFERENT RESULT Rhein 1926

Rhein ML et al. 1926 reports on root canal cases over a period of 8 years, 1918 to 1926. It is noted that his bacteriologic studies were accomplished using a culture medium of beef infusion, sheep blood agar. Thus his findings, which indicated sterility in most treated and a majority of untreated root canal cases, reflect the inability of this medium to foster growth of the actual pathogenic organism, "S. rosenow" -- in contrast to the method used by Rosenow and others who invariably then replicated Rosenow's results.

Thus Rhein's results are questionable as was his final statement, p. 981, that "It would be beneficial to the race if root-canal surgery were generally recognized as an important specialty in dentistry". Nonetheless we find him generally in support of the concept of focal infection:

"(a) The possibility of all kinds of diseases arising from dental focal infections is generally recognized.

RHEIN CLAIMS TO PRECEDE HUNTER Rhein 1926
  "(b) During the period from 1885 to 1900, when I first called attention to such a possibility, this theory was given no credence by the many medical men to whom I presented it. In fact it was generally ridiculed.
  "(c) After Hunter presented his case, the physician was converted. Losing all sense of equilibrium, many of them have gone to the extreme ...
  "(d) The pendulum is now again beginning to swing toward the median line."

HOLMAN'S TRIAL FRAUD BALLOON Holman 1927
  Holman 1927 - The buildup. In a preview of his upcoming (1928) scam, Holman in a 1927 letter to JAMA praised Rosenow et. al. for "emphasizing the importance of chronic infected foci in many types of disease", and offered that "... the issue of secondary infections arising from primary foci [is] a sequence of events, the main features of which are largely accepted"; however, he asserted that this issue is not to be compared with that of "elective localization" which he referred to as "a theory with little if any experimental basis" [p. 434].
  Holman then proceeded to explain why he felt Rosenow's elective localization work was deficient:
  "One difficulty in accepting the results of such extensive experimental work [of Rosenow and his co-workers] as convincing evidence of acquired specific tissue affinity of the streptococci used is that we do not agree on a premise. Should we not take as our basis for discussion the experimental production of the lesions or localization being considered, and then determine the percentage of these results brought about by the so-called specific and non-specific strains? From this point of view the earlier work of Rosenow, on which the theory is founded, does not indicate more than a 50% chance for either 'specific' or 'non-specific' strains. There are slight variations on both sides of this middle point, but they are not significant and can be explained on the basis of experimental error."[p.435]
  BUT, REMEMBERING THAT THIS "50%" IS THE NONSENSE EXPOSED ABOVE IN <2> "THE FACTS", HOW CAN WE NOT BE UP IN ARMS OVER THE ERROR OF ITS ACCEPTANCE BY REIMANN AND HAVENS AND THE ENTIRE FOUNDING GENERATION OF ROOT-CANAL "THERAPY" ADVOCATES, ITS ADOPTION AT FACE VALUE BY INTERNAL MEDICINE DOYEN BEESON, AND OVERALL ITS HAVING BEEN FOISTED ON THE REST OF MEDICINE, AND ON US - THEIR GUINEA PIGS?

HOLMAN'S FRAUDULENT PACKAGE WAS HEFTY (69 pp.) Holman 1928
  Although Rosenow, in articles subsequent to both Holman and Reimann /Havens articles, responded to all other points and also provided supportive data from additional studies, he appears to not have directly addressed Holman's fraudulent statistical presentation.
  Holman 1928 - pp. 68-136, begins with the sentence: "Focal infection has changed, with increased evidence from a theory to a principle of infection.", and concludes that "Focal infection is a

principle of great importance in numerous disease conditions in man", but nonetheless asserts, "I think it is evident that streptococci can cause certain lesions throughout the animal body, but that it is roughly a 50 per cent chance whether any particular localization occurs with a 'specific' or 'non-specific' strain." ...

   "The conclusion to be drawn from the reports available is that elective localization as a hypothesis to explain the occurrence and incidence of focal infection as it is found in man is insufficient.
  However, what Rosenow and his followers particularly showed and what all the other investigators of the problem have definitely demonstrated is that streptococci do localize in various organs and tissues and can produce lesions at least sufficiently suggestive of those found in man so that their potential danger in infected foci cannot be neglected. ... " (Billings would later, in 1938 in JAMA, point out the inherent inconsistency of this para.)

   Holman's eager followers proceeded to build an anti-focal-infection "church" upon Holman's deception:

HOLMAN'S LEGACY PERPETUATED MacNevin 1930
   MacNevin 1930 - The concluding pages (p. 88-89) of his chapter on "The Mechanism of Oral Focal Infection" duplicates Holman's arguments against Rosenow, largely in quotes and commencing with Holman's statement that "it is roughly a 50 per cent. chance whether any particular localization occurs with a 'specific' or 'non-specific' strain." Nonetheless, Tellier in MacNevin 30, p. 238, states: "Many apparently unexplainable post operative deaths may result from carious teeth."
   It is particularly notable that except where MacNevin relies on Holman, and to some extent even where he does, MacNevin is supportive of the Rosenow position.
   MacNevin 1930, p. 78, cites Holman 1928: "Focal infection is a principle of infection of great importance in numerous disease conditions in man."
   p. 82, MacNevin notes that "the mouth is an especially favorable site for the development of foci of infection."
   p. 88-9, Virtually all of the last 1-1/2 pages of 8 total pages in "Chapter IV, The Mechanism of Focal Infection"; and the last 1-1/2 of 2 pages on elective localization are quoted from Holman.

HIPPOCRATES ON ORAL SEPSIS   MacNevin 1930
   MacNevin 1930 cites Hippocrates on the effects of oral sepsis on adjacent areas (nasal, oral, and throat disease, Chapter 5), ear infection (Chapter 6), eyes (Chapter 7) [Galen 150 AD called the canine teeth 'eye teeth' "because they were supplied by a branch of the optic nerve"], malignancy in the mouth (Chapter 8), digestive system (Ch. 10), circulatory and hematopoietic systems (Ch. 11).
   p. 238, "The importance of removing all possible sources of infection from the mouth and throat before operations on the gastro-intestinal tract has been stressed by Tellier [1931], Andresen and others."

MacNevin 1930, p. 388
"One group of workers claims that it is impossible to sterilize the pulp canal and dentine. ... the tooth may still contain a sufficient number of bacteria which continually pass into the system and give rise to focal infection. ...

"Black found that 45% of a series of teeth with root canal fillings were abscessed. The percentage for poor fillings was 63% and for good fillings 9%. Hyatt reports ... 41% for poor fillings and 25% for good fillings. Hadley and Rickert state that approximately 1/2 of teeth with filled root canals and 3/4 of those with unfilled canals are infected."

p. 389, MacNevin 1930 cites numerous studies since the turn of the century which show that predominating organisms in the bacteriology of infected pulps are streptococci, primarily alpha type (viridans).

WRONG PROCEDURE BUT SUPPORTS ROSENOW   Valentine and van Meter 1930
Valentine and Van Meter - While Appleton would in 1933 (see below) refer to Valentine and Van Meter as having contradicted Rosenow, and as Rosenow has pointed out, they did not follow proper culture methodology, their results nonetheless uniformly showed a percentage of localization consistently higher in animals inoculated with cultures derived from persons "with systemic diseases" as compared with that for persons without systemic disease.

TABLE 5:   LOCALIZATION IN ANIMALS - Valentine and van Meter 1930
Percentages of localization in animals with organism from infected
      <u>teeth</u> of 11 adults with systemic disease vs. 9 adults without.
Source: adults with (S) or without (N) systemic infection:

	% of animals with lesions in indicated organ	% of animals with positive S. cultures in indicated organ
	S/N	S/N
--muscle tissue	37/31	
--joints	68/63	68/63
--heart	37/10	68/26
--kidney	18/16	62/42
--brain	50/13	50/40
--lung		56/21
--spleen		68/26
--liver tissues		25/10

In the case of inoculum from the tonsils of 20 adults, 11 with systemic disease and 9 without, both lesions and positive cultures were noted in 63 vs. 50 percent of the respective groups.

Overall: Valentine and Van Meter inject only two animals per specimen, do not utilize the proper culture technic described by Rosenow & Haden etc., and in their narrative somewhat disqualify their own work from the outset with the statement "it is deemed unjustifiable to draw conclusions [involving] the injection of less than a considerable number of animals per specimen."

The authors do not discuss "systemic diseases" in detail but merely state "since the chief systemic infection in the original host was reported as arthritis or rheumatism, it is possible that the slight differences in percentages between the lesions produced in animals inoculated with material from these cases and the lesions from normal cases are significant.".

HOLMAN'S LEGACY PERPETUATED   Blayney 1932

Blayney 32 - Holman is the initial reference and portions of his conclusions are closely paraphrased, including his statement "focal infection is a principle of ... great importance" and his suggestion that "The cure of a patient after removal or treatment of a suspected focus ... may be due to ... the removal of one cause of a lowered systemic resistance."

Blayney 1932, p. 635, thus asserts "improved physical conditions following the removal of a suspected focus" do not conclusively mean that the focus was responsible initially, and then goes on to say that "it is impossible to prove a definite relationship between dental infection and systemic disorders."

Thus Blayney is now free to concentrate on the techniques of root canal therapy, which topic constitutes the bulk of his article and thus his apparent purpose in any case.

HOLMAN'S LEGACY PERPETUATED   Appleton 1933

Appleton 1933, p. 565-77: In Chapter 31, "Focal Infection", it is noted that Holman is the first (p. 566) and last citation (p. 577) in Appleton's Chapter 31, "Focal Infection"; and is also given the last outside word in a section therein entitled "Elective Tissue Affinity".

p. 565, Appleton 1933 acknowledges that "The concept of focal infection has become the most powerful single factor at work in directing dental thought and practice in the past 20 years."

p. 565, concedes that "... chronic infection about the teeth, even though the patient be aware of no discomfort, does at times insidiously result in serious and even fatal lesions in other parts of the body."

p. 574-6, section on "Elective Tissue Affinity" cites Valentine and Van Meter, who as Rosenow has noted varied in culture technique from that required and thus cannot be cited as negating Rosenow; and cites primarily Holman's conclusion that "the evidence favoring elective localization is so open to misinterpretation and so limited in its practical application that it cannot be considered as a help in the solution of the problem."

p. 577, Appleton closes his chapter on focal infection with "The most comprehensive and critical analysis of the whole subject of focal infection which has yet appeared in English is that by:

Holman: *Arch. Path.*, 1928, 5, 68."

REIGN OF TERROR OF BILLINGS/ROSENOW   Sharp 1937
   Sharp 1937, p. 1231, refers to W. D. Miller in 1891 as having
"first directed the attention of the medical and dental professions
to the relationship between infections of the mouth and many
general constitutional diseases."

ADA EDITOR JOHNSON'S MISREPRESENTATION OF HUNTER   Sharp 1937
   Sharp 1937 cites the work of William Hunter of England which
popularized the theory. Sharp cites C.N. Johnson has having
pointed out that Hunter "was concerned with the visible infection -
never with infection from the apices of the roots of teeth, the
conclusion to which the overhasty jumped." Ironically this follows
Sharp's seemingly contradictory acknowledgment that Hunter had in
fact asserted that dental work built on or around diseased teeth
"formed a veritable mausoleum of gold over a mass of sepsis", which
non-visible sepsis was clearly a prime object of Hunter's concern.

ORIGINS OF ROOT CANAL THERAPY Sharp 1937
   Sharp 1937 refers to Bourdet 1757 and Hudson 1809 as having
extirpated pulps and filled roots of anterior teeth to the apex
with gold, and Woofendale as having experimented with treating the
dental pulp in 1783. Around 1825, Flagg and Koeker used various
means of treating the pulp, including oil of cloves, oil of
cajuput, camphor, opium, alum and myrrh. In 1836 Spooner advocated
the use of arsenic to devitalize pulps; in 1839 Harris warned
against this, but his warning was ignored. John Hunter in 1835
advocated burning the nerve with acids and strong alkalies; Bell
suggested burning it with a white-hot cauterizing wire. In the mid
1850s it was common to destroy and extirpate pulps by driving a
sharp stick into the canal, but this caused many fractures and
hence the practice was ended.

SHOTGUN HISTORY OF ROOT-FILLING FAILURES   Sharp 1937
   Gutta percha was introduced as a temporary stopping around 1847,
and gutta percha root canal points were introduced in 1887. Tomes
1897 reported favorably on paraffin as a root filling.
   Witzel 1873 claimed calcification and regeneration at the apical
region of teeth whose roots had been treated and partly filled.
   During the late 1800s various substances were used for cleaning
out the canals, including creosote, creosote and arsenic, nitrate
of silver and chloride of soda, chloride of zinc, sodium and
potassium, and sulfuric acid. W.D. Miller introduced the use of a
mummifying paste in about 1893.
   Following the introduction of the use of X-rays in dentistry
around 1900, Rhein in 1911 is credited with first applying its use
to root canal work. Following this, Percy Howe advocated a silver
reduction method of treating root canals.
   All of the foregoing led Rhein to claim, "up to the time of
Hunter and Billings and Rosenow and since, much definite progress
has been made in perfecting the root-filling technic."

Whereas, the very accounting of the shotgun history of root-filling failures might have more properly led to a characterization of "absolutely no progress has been made...".

HOLMAN'S LEGACY PERPETUATED Sharp 1937
"Then Billings (1912) and Rosenow (1915) began their animal experiments in oral infection which, though not verified by the subsequent investigation of other scientific men, inaugurated a reign of terror for the pulpless tooth."
Totally ignoring all published and readily available work supportive of Rosenow, Billings et al., Sharp makes his case by mentioning or quoting no less than 13 persons who share his views [p. 1233-6] but gives only one specific reference, i.e. MacNevin and Vaughn's book. As discussed above, MacNevin's work, in turn, when it does not support focal infection, relies on Holman to reject the magnificent refinement of elective localization.
p. 1234, Sharp implies that Rosenow's work was fraudulent:
"Rosenow's spectacular experiments were, by this time [1930], being investigated by bacteriologists both in this country and abroad. Other investigators were not able to reproduce his results, and the experimental work upon which his theories are based is now widely criticized severely both in this country and in Europe."

GROSSMAN: ON THE HOLMAN BANDWAGON, FROM 1940
Grossman 1940 bases his case on Holman 1928, and on the three derivative works, MacNevin 1930, Blayney 1932 and Appleton 1933. See Grossman 1946 for more detailed discussion.

HOLMAN'S LEGACY PERPETUATED Reimann 1940
Reimann and Havens 40 - On: "the problem of elective localization of bacteria", Holman is the first of cited authors and discussion of his "review" of Rosenow's data comprises the bulk of a section on "Inoculation Experiments" (p. 1). Reimann and Havens repeat Holman's assertions that the theory of elective localization is "open to misinterpretation" and "limited in its practical application"; they then substitute the weasel-worded phrase "focal infection as herein referred" for the term "elective localization" in Holman's already-faulty assertion that elective localization had not been proved, thus paving the way for Beeson 1976 and others to disown wholly the concept of focal infection.
However, it may be noted that even Reimann and Havens, who largely ignored the successes of the focal infection concept [per Slocumb 1941], conceded that examples of improvement from systemic disease after removal of foci "suggest... an etiologic relationship."
Reimann-Havens have bought the Holman "rearrangement" fraud, hook-line-and sinker; at first the writer was inclined to attribute this to laziness, stupidity, or party to a grand conspiracy for which a case might be made as having been orchestrated by Grossman.
 As will become abundantly clear in a review of the early *JADA*,

these later folks seem to have been by then just going along with the flow. [See APPENDIX G: JADA - THE EARLY YEARS]

HOLMAN LEGACY PERPETUATED Woods 1942
  Woods 42 (ophthalmology) - Holman's views are summarized in detail (1426-7), including verbatim restatement of his sleazy "50% chance" misleading statement, as per below. Woods does add, however, "From the practical viewpoint the wisest course in the treatment and diagnosis of endogenous ocular disease is to continue the search for foci of infection."
  Woods 1942, p. 1423, notes that the modern concept of focal infection was introduced by William Hunter in 1901 [*Oral Sepsis as a Cause of Disease*, N.Y., Cassell and Co. 1901] and "elaborated chiefly by [Frank] Billings from 1910 to 1916."
  Woods 1942, p. 1427, on elective localization: " ... the elective localization of bacteria, held by many as sufficient cause in itself to account for the localization of focal infection, was held by Holman to not have been confirmed. ... While Holman conceded that a general bacteriologic adaptation of environment is universally accepted and cannot be denied, and while it is clearly proved that streptococci can cause various lesions throughout the body, nevertheless, it is a 50% chance whether any particular localization occurs with a 'specific' or 'nonspecific' strain." [Thus does Woods swallow Holman, hook-line-and-sinker, particularly "line"]
  p. 1428, Woods 1942 refers to Reimann and Havens' "well-documented review [which] ably summarized" the opposition to the position that oral focal relate to other disease conditions.
  "Far from being of benefit to the patient, the extraction of teeth may be positively dangerous, the bacteria being actually forced into the bloodstream by the trauma of operation." [this seems to be supportive of the Rosenow position]
  Following a discussion of Reimann and Havens' article, Woods concludes with the false statement, the only basis for which must be Holman's fraud, that: "The results of inoculation experiments with organisms isolated from infected teeth are all sharply in contradiction to Rosenow's experiments, and these views on elective localization, which form such a cornerstone for the focal infection theory, should not only be disregarded but actively counteracted."
  Woods 1942, p. 1431, "[The] mass of clinical evidence ... illustrating the recovery of the diseased eye on removal of foci of infection, is so formidable that it is difficult to dismiss it lightly on the sole grounds that it is only suggestive evidence."
  p. 1441 "... practically all the actual evidence in favor of the [focal infection] theory as originally set forth and generally subscribed to, is totally clinical, largely suggestive, and circumstantial. [This blatantly ignores bacteriological a la Rosenow] ... However, it is assumed that there may be a cause-and-effect relationship between a primary focus of infection and ocular disease through such a mechanism as sensitization and intoxication of the diseased eye by bacterial products absorbed from the focus of infection; a fair experimental basis can be

advanced for such an assumption, although clinical evidence is
lacking."

HOLMAN'S LEGACY PERPETUATED Crowley 1946
   J. Crowley, 1946, states "Reimann and Havens in 1940 published
an article which thoroughly reviews the literature on focal
infection ..." and goes on to quote their negative conclusion.
Crowley also refers to Woods (1942), Grossman (1940) on the
negative side, and Slocumb, et al.. (1941) on the positive.

UVEAL DISEASE Crowley 1946
   Crowley 1946 quotes Woods, "it is an established procedure to
search for foci of infection in the study of the etiology of uveal
tract disease."

ARTHRITIS/IRITIS Crowley 1946
   p. 129, Notwithstanding a recent "swing away from the general
acceptance of the theory of focal infection ..., it would be just
as serious a mistake for the dentist not to eliminate dental
infection in patients suffering from rheumatoid arthritis and
iritis."

ENDODONTIST GURU CLEARLY DECEPTIVE Grossman 1946
   Grossman 46 cites the same references as he had in 1940, plus
Reimann /Havens 1940.   [See Appendix F - THE GROSSMAN FILE, for
detailed discussions.

HOLMAN'S LEGACY PERPETUATED Wolfson 1949
   Wolfson, 1949, cites prominently the conclusions of Burket,
Woods, Grossman, and McNevin and Vaughn.
   Wolfson 1949 concludes with a quote from McNevin and Vaughn:
"that the proofs submitted by Price and Rosenow and others had
their limitations from the standpoints of both technique and
interpretation of results." In other words, they prefer Holman's
math.

WHAT LEFT OF FOCAL INFECTION THEORY? "A GOOD DEAL!" Kern, 1950
BOIL & NEPHRITIS Kern, 1950
   Kern, 1950, asks: "What is left of the theory of focal
infection?" and concludes "a good deal".
   p. 1706, "a boil on the back of the neck is at times followed by
a perinephritic abscess.
   p. 1707, cites importance of conditioning factors in disease,
whereby "the focus only rarely appears as the sole factor."
   p. 1708, points out fallacies in the arguments against focal
infection;
   p. 1710, lists practical considerations including: "Dental,
tonsillar and prostatic foci comprise the great majority of those
with major significance"; and "A focus of infection when found
deserves treatment"
   Cites Grossman's conservative principles concerning management of
pulpless teeth, e.g., where bone is destroyed equal to 1/3 of the

root surface, where crown cannot be restored, or one with an area
of rarefaction where focal infection is suspected.
    p. 1711, cites "The commonest diseases in which a relationship to
a focus of infection deserves serious consideration are: infectious
arthritis, iritis, iridocyclitis, bacterial endocarditis, acute
glomerulonephritis, myositis and neuritis."
    p. 1712, "Each piece of evidence, proved or circumstantial, in
support of the theory can be found as admitted by one or the other
of nearly every one of those who opposed it. There is something
left of the theory of focal infection; a good deal."

FOCAL INFECTION DEFINED Easlick 1951
    p. 618, "A focus of infection is a circumscribed and confined
area that contains pathogenic micro-organisms and that usually
causes no clinical manifestations [citing Kronfeld 1939]. The
development of secondary lesions, traceable to this primary focus,
constitutes focal infection." [citing Appleton 1944]

FOCAL INFECTION FIRMLY ESTABLISHED Easlick 1951
    p. 619, "A careful review of the literature permits the
investigator to conclude that focal infection operates through the
transmission of bacteria by the blood or lymph circulation."
    p. 619, cites Reimann and Havens 1940: "The concept of focal
infection in relation to systemic disease is firmly established."
    p. 621, the section "Scientific support of elective localization"
is inextricably dependent on Holman 1928, Grossman 1940 and Woods,
on the subject of elective localization.

HOLMAN'S LEGACY PERPETUATED Easlick 1951
    p. 621, "In 1928 Holman reviewed the literature critically and
commented on the theory of elective localization: 'The specificity
of the bacteria has not been proved and the theory of elective
localization is so open to misinterpretation and so limited in its
practical application that it cannot be considered as a help in the
solution of the problem.' ..." [Same section was cited verbatim by
others, e.g., Appleton 1933, Grossman 1946.]

RHEUMATIC FEVER AND TEETH   Easlick 1951
    Easlick et al., *JADA* 42 (June 1951), p. 623] report that Denny et
al.. found a reduced attack rate of rheumatic fever by the
treatment of streptococcic disease with penicillin. Two of 798
treated patients, v. 12 of 804 untreated, developed acute rheumatic
fever. "This finding appears highly significant, since such a
difference could be due to chance only 6 in 10,000 times. Easlick
p. 631, also refers to Taran cites higher prevalence of tooth decay
in children with or having had rheumatic fever; Stein of Vienna and
Rolleston have observed a higher incidence of rheumatic fever in
children suffering from dental infections than with healthy teeth.
    Easlick et al., 1951, p. 627-8, in a search for the source of
streptococci concerned in subacute bacterial endocarditis, noted
that "a transient streptococcal bacteremia lasting a few minutes

was observed [after tooth extractions] in 75% of the cases [138 patients] considered to exhibit a severe type of oral sepsis, and in 34% of the patients with no obvious gum disease." These were S. viridans in the majority of cases.

   p. 630, "It may be concluded that ample evidence is available to show that transient bacteremias follow the extraction of teeth."

   p. 643, Easlick cites a study of 632 root canal cases in which the presence of pain seemed to have little bearing on whether or not positive bacteriologic cultures were obtained, i.e., of cases with a history of no pain, 49.9% yielded positive cultures, v. 52.5% of cases exhibiting mild pain and 55.3% of cases experiencing severe pain.

VASCULAR HEART DISEASE, BLOOD Easlick 1951
   Easlick 1951, p. 663, note that Kinsella proposed that "The nonhemolytic streptococcus is responsible for 90-95% of the cases of this type of endocarditis [subacute bacterial] ... The gonococcus is responsible in the remaining 5-10%.

   p. 670, "This was confirmed by Friedberg, who stated in 1949 that 95% of cases of subacute bacterial endocarditis are caused by nonhemolytic streptococci. ... It has been repeatedly noted that subacute bacterial endocarditis develops following the extraction of a tooth or removal of tonsils. ... The S. viridans is the common organism found in infected tonsils and dental apical abscesses and may be thrust into the bloodstream by operative procedures."

   p. 683, "It is well to note that by far the most frequent organisms cultivated from non-vital teeth are viridans and nonhemolytic streptococci. ...

   "There appears to be little evidence to link the activity of these two common organisms in teeth with manifestations of disease in the integument." [Thus does Easlick write off Rosenow and fact.]

HIPPOCRATES ON FOCAL INFECTION Kolmer 1952
   p. 141, Kolmer includes as primary dental infections (and presumable foci of infection) infected impacted teeth (especially the third molar) which is reminiscent of Hippocrates's statement, as per MacNevin 1930, p. 92: "Hippocrates (460 BC) said that 'Suppurations arising from the third tooth are more frequent than from any other; and the dense discharge from the nose, and pains in the temple, are especially owing to it."

   p. 146-7, on elective localization:
   "A number of pathogenic bacteria display an affinity or elective localization for particular organs or tissues, such as the predominant tendency of meningococci to infect the meninges, gonococci the urethra and adnexa and pneumococci the respiratory tract. It is not necessary for physicians and dentists to assume that streptococci, staphylococci or other microorganisms in primary foci of infection acquire a selective affinity for this or that organ or tissue as postulated by Rosenow [*Internat. Clin.* 2:29 (June) 1930]. Indeed this theory of elective localization has been

largely if not entirely abandoned. Abandoning the theory, however, does not detract from the important principles of focal infection in the etiology of systemic diseases. Rather, it appears that there are other factors which determine the secondary localization of infection [e.g.] ... altering of the endothelium of capillaries with reduction in circulation, [and] ... the possibility of vascular changes due to heredity tending to capillary occlusion, especially in the etiology of rheumatoid arthritis."

Kolmer offers that this would explain why some people with prominent foci escape diseases potentially due to such foci, whereas others with minor primary foci develop such diseases.

BLOOD, ANEMIA, ANOREXIA, CHRONIC FATIGUE SYNDROME Kolmer 1952
p. 147, "It is reasonable to assume that such general conditions as anemia, anorexia, or fatigability, may be due to the production and absorption of exogenous or endogenous bacterial toxins or other toxic products in primary foci of infection ...

"It is also possible, and highly probable, as originally stated by Billings, that acquired hypersensitivity to bacteria or their soluble products in the primary foci of infection plays a role in the genesis of the secondary lesions of focal infection. If this is true one must assume that the bacteria or their products reach secondary foci by way of the blood."

p. 149, "... it may be stated that at least one mechanism in the production of the secondary diseases of focal infection is the occurrence of transient periods of bacteremia".

"As stated by Kern [1950], every farmer knows that lighting matches in a barn is a real hazard, although the number escaping damage or destruction exceeds the number burning down, so likewise primary foci of infection may produce ill health only in some individuals."

SYMPTOMLESS FOCI - DANGER Kolmer 1952
"Paradoxically ... foci presenting the minimum of inflammatory changes are potentially the more dangerous. Inflammation produces a nonspecific resistance by arresting the spread of bacteria" through a number of ways.

p. 151, "There can be no doubt about the importance of specific natural antibodies and phagocytosis as well."

p. 152, Kolmer lists numerous diseases definitely or possibly resulting from focal infection, including those due to septicemias, bacteremias or toxemias, lymphogenous infections, direct continuity and acquired allergic sensitization.

RHEUMATOID ARTHRITIS Kolmer 1952
"That [rheumatoid arthritis] is a systemic disease and not a disease of the joints alone is indicated by the presence of unusual cardiac lesions which occur in some individuals." Kolmer cites Hench's "impressive though not conclusive" evidence that it is at least in part due to focal infection."

p. 153, Kolmer discusses the treatment of conditions and diseases due to focal infection:

(1) eradication of primary foci of infection. This is "not likely to be of benefit in rheumatoid arthritis of one or more years' duration."

NEGATIVE ROOT CANAL CULTURES Kolmer 1952
   p. 154, Some dentists "doubt the value of negative root canal cultures because of the possible presence of pathogenic microorganisms in the dentinal tubules, which eventually makes extraction necessary. ...

ENDOCARDITIS Kolmer 1952
   " In a grave disease such as subacute bacterial endocarditis, primary foci should never be disturbed until the patient is fully protected by adequate antibiotic therapy, and, in the case of infected teeth, only one or two should be extracted at a time."

VACCINE THERAPY Kolmer 1952
   Kolmer 1952, p. 155, states that it is not surprising that vaccine therapy has been largely abandoned due to all the abuses in preparation and administration. Kolmer relates his own experience of the previous 40 years "exclusively with autogenous vaccines [which] have proved sufficiently satisfactory to include them in therapeutic programs, particularly in the treatment of chronic recurrent iritis and other ocular diseases, intrinsic asthma, fibrositis (especially in myositis, perineuritis or bursitis), and in rheumatoid arthritis. ... In the great majority of instances the vaccines have been prepared of viridans streptococci alone or in combination with coagulase positive staphylococci."

ENDOCARDITIS, SUBACUTE BACTERIAL Kolmer 1952
   Kolmer 1952, p. 157, regarding subacute bacterial endocarditis, "... dentists have a special responsibility since so many instances of the disease may be traced to focal infection of dental origin. Physicians should not only see to it that all patients with rheumatic, hypertensive and other types of valvular and congenital heart disease receive periodic dental care but also that the dentists concerned are informed of the existence of these types of heart disease in their patients. ...
   "If in doubt it appears far better to extract a tooth, or teeth, than to take chances on subacute bacterial endocarditis or some other grave disease of focal infection, not only because 'an empty house is better than a poor tenant' but because of the present high excellence of restorative dentistry. Furthermore, it is always advisable to extract only one or two teeth at a time, in order to reduce the chances of transient bacteremia."

PENDULUM SWINGING TOO FAR FROM FOCAL INFECTION Kolmer 1952
   Kolmer 1952, p. 158 Discussion and Conclusions: "... focal infection in the etiology of various systemic diseases is no longer a theory but a process or mechanism well established in both medicine and dentistry. ... It is ... fortunate that the era of 'focal infection delirium' with the wholesale and needless

extractions of teeth or removal of tonsils has at least largely passed .... On the other hand, the pendulum of opinion may be swinging too far in the opposite direction with unwarranted skepticism on the potential clinical importance of focal infection in the etiology of disease."

Kolmer 1952, p. 159, "Since the microorganisms of focal infection are usually of reduced virulence, a high incidence of escape from ill health is both inevitable and expected."

Kolmer states that reports that have minimized "the potential importance of focal infections in relation to rheumatoid arthritis, uveitis and other diseases" are based largely on the observation that foci may be as common in healthy persons as in sick ones, whereas as stated above hereditary factors are also operative.

FOCAL INFECTION CANNOT BE DISCARDED JAMA 1952

Editorial *JAMA* 1952, p. 490, notes that "the theory of focal infection in the past 10 or 15 years has fallen in part into disfavor. This has been partly due to the excesses and abuses that have been committed in its name, and partly to the following observations that seem to discredit it. (1) Many patients with diseases presumably caused by foci of infection have not been relieved of their symptoms by removal of the foci. (2) Many patients with these same systemic diseases have no evident focus of infection. (3) Foci of infection are, according to some statistical studies, as common in apparently healthy persons as in those with disease.

"... none of [these] actually disprove the theory ... (1) This does not prove ... that the focus did not initiate the disease [or that] undiscovered foci are not responsible for its maintenance"; "(2) ... does not prove the absence of concealed foci ... [or] that a mechanism similar to focal infection is not operative in these cases, as [in] a temporary bacteriemia"; "(3) ... only proves that foci alone, with accessing factors ... are not sufficient. Thus on logical grounds alone the basic theory cannot be discarded."

"In positive support of a modified theory of focal infection is the fact that certain foci are known to be capable of producing disseminated disease. Kolmer supplies a long list of such foci and diseases in an extensive review", which included acute bacterial endocarditis, osteomyelitis, suppurative myelitis, perirenal abscess, acute rheumatic fever and other systemic manifestations. Kolmer concluded "that the etiological role of focal infection in some systemic diseases is no longer theory, but fact."

"In view of the demonstrated importance of foci of infection in some diseases, and the still valid theoretical possibility that they contribute to the production of others, it is apparent that focal infection cannot be ignored in the practice of medicine. ...

In early disease [in patients with diseases known to be due to focal infection] eradication of foci may relieve symptoms; in advanced disease it should not be expected to do so, although it may lighten the load on the body's adaptive capacities."

HOLMAN'S LEGACY PERPETUATED Easlick 1953
   Easlick 1953, p. 180, cites Holman 1928: "It is now realized, in spite of the evident adaptation of some bacteria to a specific environment, that the validity of the theory of elective localization of bacteria has not been demonstrated."
   Easlick totally ignores Rosenow and Billings, etc., while paraphrasing Holman and quoting Grossman (sections which are based largely on Holman) and Reimann, etc.
   p. 182, Easlick warns of the "possibility of local extension of an oral infection, or invasion of the blood stream.
   "Dentists appear to have sufficient information to warrant particular concern about oral surgical intervention or the presence of oral foci in the mouths of patients with valvular heart disease.
    S. viridans ... most frequently are associated with subacute bacterial endocarditis ... .
   p. 183, "... the final scientific appraisal by the modern dentist of the role of oral foci in human disease demands a critical approach to available information." [A TRULY CRITICAL APPROACH DEMANDS CESSATION OF ROOT-CANAL "THERAPY"]

HOLMAN LEGACY PERPETUATED; HYPOCRITICAL OATH Jawetz 1955
   Jawetz's negatively-toned discussion draws heavily on McNevin and Vaughn (1924).
   Jawetz 1955, p. 1063, suggests, that given the passage of time since the major era of controversy between medicine and dentistry that "it may be possible to examine the problem from a detached standpoint and in a dispassionate mood and to attempt to assess its role in the rational management of patients."

BILLINGS AS EXHORTER Jawetz 1955
ROSENOW AS ADDING "A TOUCH OF REFINEMENT" Jawetz 1955
   Jawetz refers to Billings as initiating the conflict by "exhorting the relationship between 'oral sepsis' and a variety of physical and mental illnesses ... . This theory was given a touch of refinement by Rosenow's doctrine of 'selective affinity' ... [whereby] a streptococcus from the tooth of a person with duodenal ulcer would locate by preference in the duodenum of an animal into which it was injected. A good deal of effort was expended in trying to document this strange and wonderful mechanism - alas with success in the hands of only a very few particularly gifted (or prejudiced?) investigators." [This one {Jawetz} should have been pilloried at least].
   Notwithstanding this less-than-objective start, Jawetz nonetheless discusses how transient oral bacteria might cause endocarditis or small abscesses in kidney, glomeruli or synovial membranes. He also discusses how hypersensitivity associated with oral sepsis may play a role in producing iritis, arthritis or other conditions, which may be "helped or even cured by the removal of a tooth abscess." Jawetz devotes much space to the need for prophylaxis and treatment of systemic disease originating from 'focal infection' of the oral cavity ..."

MOUTH INFECTIONS, VIRAL INFECTIONS Jawetz 1955, p. 1069
"In many viral infections, oral lesions occur principally very
early in the disease, at the end of the incubation period, or
during the prodromal stage which precedes the typical symptoms of
the disease. Outstanding examples are the mouth lesions of the
infectious diseases of childhood, such as measles and chicken pox.
..."

POLIO CORRELATED WITH TONSILLITIS Jawetz 1955
  "Infection with herpes simplex virus gives prominent oral
manifestations during both the primary infection and the later
recurrent lesions."
  p. 1072, "The occurrence of bulbar poliomyelitis has been
definitely correlated with tonsillectomy during epidemic periods."

HOLMAN'S LEGACY PERPETUATED Coolidge 1960
  Coolidge 1960 refers to Appleton as having "enumerated many
unsolved factors [which] ... present a great challenge for future
investigation." Overall Coolidge concludes that "neither
endodontics nor the theory of focal infection have contributed
sufficient evidence for the scientific evaluation and resolution of
the problem." Nonetheless, without Appleton, who goes down with
Holman, Coolidge would have to support Rosenow.
  Coolidge notes "many questions remain unanswered.
p. 680, refers to 1890 work of W.D. Miller referring to
"decomposition of the contents of dental tubules as a disturbing
factor in the treatment of pulpless teeth", and Black's work in
1891 on the same subject.
- refers to Buckley's introduction of formocresol in 1904 as a
chemical control of gaseous products of pulp decomposition.
- Refers to Billings 1904 on oral sepsis, Rosenow 1909 on elective
localization, and "shortly after, in 1911, Dr. William Hunter of
London" on oral sepsis (whereas Hunter's work had come out
previously, in the late 19th century).
- p. 681, refers to "extreme of tooth extraction in clinical
practice, and then that "much confusion followed for two decades or
more" which was "soon explained by the impossibility of
disinfecting the surface of extracted human teeth and the
contamination of the root surface ..." as demonstrated by Fish and
MacLean and others ... "These findings discounted the importance of
many earlier reports." Thus here we see Coolidge buying into the
Grossman mentality and arguments.
- p. 682, discusses Grossman and others "who gave great support to
the idea of culturing before filling.
- p. 683, notes that "Each new drug recommended for endodontic
treatment was found to have certain limitations... Of the
combinations, Grossman's polyantibiotic formula has been widely
used since 1951 with varied reports on the advantages of its use.
- p. 684, notes "The purpose of filling root canals is to
obliterate them, or, at least, to seal the apical foramens with
inert material to prevent any inflow of tissue exudate into the
canal in which reinfection can occur. ...

- p. 685-6, states that Aguilar 1957 "has well said, 'The phenomena
of repair of the periapical region in cases of pulpless teeth and
especially with chronic periapical lesions continues, together with
the theory of focal infection, to be an object of the greatest
controversy. The reason is that neither endodontics nor the theory
of focal infection have contributed sufficient evidence for the
scientific evaluation and resolution of the problem.'"
   Coolidge cites Rosenow 1909, 1916, and 1919, nothing later; and
Hunter 1911.

HOLMAN'S LEGACY PERPETUATED; INTO THE 60s Topazian 1962
   Topazian 1962 cites Holman 1928, Grossman 1940 and Easlick 1951;
all heavily dependent on Holman's deception.
   Topazian, p. 1075, "Bacteremia following dental operations is an
unquestionable factor in the production of focal infection in cases
where certain predisposing conditions exist."
   p. 1076: "The theory of elective localization as postulated by
Rosenow ... stated that the secondary localization of bacteria
which had arrived from the primary focus was due to a specific
affinity of those bacteria for certain tissues. However, the
theory has been disproved or seriously questioned by various
reliable observers." [And who are these "reliable observers"?
Topazian cites Holman 1928, Grossman 1940 and Easlick 1951; all
heavily dependent on Holman's deception. What seems particularly
telling, beyond the continued reliance on this decades-old fraud,
is the nonexistence of any studies since that might be invoked
against Rosenow. In other words the opposition to Rosenow is
wholly lacking in foundation.]

ENDOCARDITIS Topazian 1962
   p. 1079, Topazian cites a number of studies "which definitely
incriminated dental foci of infection as serious offenders in this
disease [subacute bacterial endocarditis]
   p. 1081, "... oral foci of infection should always be removed
regardless of the physical condition of the patient, and ... foci
of infection should be removed in almost every disease process in
an attempt to increase the general health of the patient. ..."

BEESON IGNORES FOCAL INFECTION PROOFS Beeson 1963
   Beeson and McDermott 1963, p. 1479, "Any infection, evident or
'focal', should be treated by whatever means is necessary for its
eradication. It is rare indeed that a dramatic change in the
course of the disease follows the treatment of such infection, and
indiscriminate removal of teeth, tonsils and even internal organs
because they might be sites of 'focal infection' is to be
condemned." (Such indiscriminate removal was in fact also shunned
by Rosenow, etc.)

HOLMAN LEGACY IS HISTORICAL RECORD BY 1963 McManus 1963, p. 59.
   The level of general acceptance of the anti-Rosenow, anti-focal-
infection-concept view, by 1963, is evident in historian McManus's
slam-dunk, off-the-wall, pop-science mis-characterization and

rejection of the truly insidious role of Rosenow's streptococcus:
"As a warning against too readily implicating any living agent as a cause, merely because it has been found in a lesion, we need to recall the suggestions that ... the streptococcus caused a variety of diseases ranging from poliomyelitis to rheumatoid arthritis to ulcerative colitis and so on almost ad infinitum." [p. 59].

BIOFEEDBACK JUMPS ON ANTI-ROSENOW BANDWAGON McManus 1963, 65.
"To heart disease we now must add asthma, many varieties of skin diseases, various types of peptic ulceration, and a number of other condition whose psychosomatic basis is now more than suggested."
[p. 65]
It is notable that by 1990s the pendulum had decisively moved in the opposite direction, with peptic ulcers in particular now definitively believed to be caused by a "helicobacter pylori", and the correlation between heart disease and teeth newly rediscovered and firmly established.

HOLMAN'S LEGACY PERPETUATED, HERE AND EVERYWHERE Harris 1966
Harris, M., 1966, does not cite Holman 1928, but cites Woods 1942 who had repeated Holman's arguments.
Harris, 1966, discusses acute dental infection relative to cavernous sinus thrombophlebitis and orbital cellulitis; and latent dental infection, e.g., bacteriemia from tooth extraction or even mastication; and concludes that there is little objective evidence of dental infection causing diseases of the eye except for two cases of direct spread.

BILLINGS PRAISED; FOCAL INFECTION DOWNPLAYED Hirsch 1966
Hirsch 1966 notes that Frank Billings had "motivated studies on the relationship of focal infection to systemic diseases. ... Dr. Billings regarded the invitation to deliver the Lane Lectures on focal infection [as relates to systemic disease] at the Leland Stanford Jr. Medical School in San Francisco, September 20-24, 1915, as his greatest honor. For twelve or more years, according to his introduction, the study was carried out with clinical material at Rush Medical College, affiliated with the University of Chicago, and the Presbyterian Hospital. Billings aroused the interest of clinicians, the nursing staff, and the patients in his investigation and developed a cooperative team effort in the project. ... The dimensions of this project increased to where eventually the McCormick Memorial Institute for Infectious Diseases, the Ortho S.A. Sprague Memorial Institute, and the Pathological and Research Laboratories of St. Luke's Hospital participated."
Hirsch mentions many reports that were published in the *Journal of Infectious Diseases* and specifically mentions L. Hektoen, E. R. Le Count, H.G. Wells and D.J. Davis, but notably fails to mention Rosenow, whose data summary was the centerpiece of Billing's Lane Lecture Series and whose work was of central importance. D.J. Davis is referred to as an "active" participant in bacteriological studies, and is cited by Hirsch as having, in his later years,

emphasized that tissue susceptibility and not specificity of cocci
was responsible for localization in rabbits.

FOCAL THEORY "CUT DOWN TO SIZE" Norton 1969
  Norton 1969, p. 157, cites "Examples ... of theories that have
now been cut down to size, are the germ theory, allergy, and focal
sepsis."

RHEUMATOID ARTHRITIS Norton 1969
  p. 168, re rheumatoid arthritis:
  "By the 1930s, the prevailing view, supported by much evidence,
was that the disease was infective in origin and it was customary
to hunt in every case for foci of infection in teeth, sinuses,
tonsils and gall bladder or elsewhere and to eradicate them. Some
time later, largely because actual organisms could so seldom be
found in the affected joints, the focal sepsis theory was modified.
  It was suggested that either the disease was caused by toxins
absorbed from a focus of infection or that the organisms produced a
sensitization of the joint and other tissues concerned and that the
arthritis was in fact an allergic manifestation.

FOCAL INFECTION THEORY DISCARDED WITH WARM CLIMATE Norton 1969
  "... Needless to say, regimes of treatment based on ... the
eradication of septic foci, a warm climate, and special diets, all
had their successes, but for the majority they failed to cure or
even to relieve." [False, at least as pertains to septic foci; but
there seems to be no way to effectively challenge such gratuitous
and false pronouncements.]

ARTHRITIS Anderson, 1971
  Anderson, 1971, p. 289, cites Benjamin Rush's "report in 1801 of
the cure of a patient with rheumatism of the hip following
extraction of a tooth." However, Anderson reflects the general
trend to dismiss the overall concept of focal infection due to its
abuses: "It is the general opinion today that more harm than good
has resulted from the indiscriminate extraction of teeth, tonsils,
etc... ."

HOLMAN'S LEGACY PERPETUATED
  Burket 1971, p. 554, offers "The periodic authoritative reviews
of Holmans, Rieman and Havens; Eastlick et al.. [the preceding four
names were misspelled; Crowley and Seltzer; and Jawetz furnish a
good background for the proper integration of focal infection in
the practice of internal medicine".
  All five of Burket's historical references are ultimately
dependent on Holman's fraud. Nonetheless Burket does stress the
importance of oral foci (1) in complications associated with
pregnancy; (2) in diseases of the eye; and (3) as may be related to
arthritic conditions; and also lists as supporting evidence of
focal infection (1) clinical observations, (2) findings at
necropsy, and (3) laboratory studies.
  Burket 1971, p. 550, cites as evidence supporting the concept of

focal infection:
(1) Clinical studies wherein elimination of suspected foci was
followed by disappearance of remote symptoms.
(2) the common finding at necropsy of similar primary foci and
remote disease processes.
(3) laboratory studies.
   p.554 "When multiple foci are present any single focus assumes
less significance as a causative or an aggravating factor of
disease elsewhere."

PREGNANCY Burket 1971
   "Clinical studies indicate that oral foci are important factors
in many of the complications associated with pregnancy."

PULPLESS TEETH QUESTION IN 1971 PARROTS HOLMAN Burket 1971
   p. 555, "Both Grossman and Blayney have reviewed the pulpless
tooth question and have concluded that the condemnation of teeth
merely because they are pulpless has no clinical or laboratory
justification." [As noted elsewhere, both Grossman's and Blayney's
cases against pulpless teeth rely inextricably on Holman's fraud.]

OPHTHALMOLOGY Burket 1971
EYE DISEASES Burket 1971
GLAUCOMA Burket 1971
IRITIS Burket 1971
OPTIC NEURITIS Burket 1971
   Burket 1971 reviews ophthalmology, asserting that the importance
of oral foci as a cause or aggravating factor in a variety of eye
diseases as "well-recognized by ophthalmologists." So implicated
are choroiditis, chorioretinitis, keratitis, glaucoma, retrobulbar
neuritis, iritis, iridocyclitis, episcleritis, tenonitis and some
forms of optic neuritis.
   p. 555-6, "Spaeth believes that intraocular surgery should not be
performed, except in cases of real emergency, until all dental foci
have been eliminated. Repeated clinical observations have proved
the correctness of this observation."

ARTHRITIS Burket 1971
   p. 556 "If an exacerbation of symptoms should be experienced
following the extraction of teeth or gingival curettage, it should
be regarded as highly suggestive of an etiologic relation between
the dental focus and the affected joints. ...
   "Clinical improvement following the elimination of oral foci may
not occur even when dental foci are of etiologic significance. Too
frequently the patient seeks medical advice late in the course of
the disease when secondary foci have already been established."

HOLMAN'S VIEW ENSHRINED AS BALANCE TO ROSENOW DiStefano 1971
   DiStefano, 1971, p. 245, refers to both Rosenow and Holman, in a
single sentence, the former as having implicated microorganisms in
focal infection as harmful by virtue of their affinity for
particular tissues, and the latter as harmful owing to their

causing a diminished local resistance; but DiStefano does not appear to cast the latter as a "spoiler" for the former's work. No specific Holman reference is given, whereas Rosenow is specifically cited [*Am. Dent. Surg.*, 1927]

p. 246-7, lists several diseases which may be related to dental foci, elaborating on various dermatoses.

HOLMAN'S LEGACY PERPETUATED AT BI-CENTENNIAL:

Beeson & Grossman Take Their Shots:

HOLMAN'S LEGACY PERPETUATED BIG-TIME IN MEDICINE Beeson 1976
In celebrating the demise of "the focal infection fad", Beeson turns to Reimann and Havens 1940 as having struck the "decisive blow". Yet even Beeson's referential ancestors (Reimann and Havens, 1940, and Holman, 1928) would have reprimanded him for his blanket, simplistic dismissal of the whole of the concept of focal infection.
Beeson 1976, p. 151:   "The clinical record of the U.S., although generally good during the present century, contains one entry in which we can take little satisfaction: the doctrine of focal infection and systemic disease. ... The focal infection fad had its beginnings with a paper published in 1912 by Frank Billings of Chicago. ... who later served as president of the A.M.A. ... He ... relied primarily on collaboration with the bacteriologist Edward C. Rosenow of the Mayo Clinic. ... By 1915 the focal infection craze was in full flower ... [p. 152] ... Over a 30 year period literally millions of unnecessary surgical and dental procedures were carried out in vain efforts to alleviate a larger variety of disorders. ... The decisive blow against this practice was a critical review by Hobart A. Reimann and W. Paul Havens in 1940."
As indicated above, Reimann and Havens had fundamentally relied on Holman 1928 as having "dealt with" Rosenow's claim to have demonstrated elective localization of bacteria in laboratory experiments.
It is noted that Beeson was a decade late on the Billings AMA Presidency (1902), which had preceded his work with Rosenow on focal infection. We are again reminded Beeson at the time was considered to be the "doyen" of American internal medicine (Reines, Nature 1989), so that his views on focal infection would not only reflect but also substantially influence the medical climate. Given his position within medicine and his own statements on Rosenow, Beeson was clearly aware of the solidity of Rosenow's work and its effect on all of internal medicine. Thus Beeson's attempt to pass off all of focal infection as a "craze" might even be viewed from the perspective of a "turf" war over the field of internal medicine, and an indication of how this misinformation has become entrenched in the foundations of modern medicine.

GROSSMAN'S BI-CENTENNIAL SHOW Grossman 1976
Grossman, in his Bi-Centennial overview of the field, discounted Parreidt's 1889 description of the concept of focal infection as

"an old theory rediscovered"; downplayed Hunter's well-publicized work early in the century that popularized the notion that pulpless teeth are a health hazard; poked fun at laboratory studies; and asserted that the focal-infection- concept's "death knell was sounded by controlled clinical studies". No specific references are cited, but when his earlier works are consulted, all roads lead back to Holman.
   [See also APPENDIX C, para. C and APPENDIX F on Grossman 1976.]

HOLMAN'S LEGACY PERPETUATED Bellizzi and Cruse 1980
   Bellizi and Cruse 1980 - In this heavily slanted attack, the authors contrast the "focal infection era" (1909-1937) with "the scientific era" of 1937-1962.
   Bellizzi and Cruse 1980, p. 576, refer to advocates of the focal infection theory "who condemned all pulpless teeth to extraction" and the "one-hundred percenters" who "followed the whims and directions of the medical profession."
   B & C refer to E.C. Rosenow as "Charles" Rosenow, whereas the C. in E.C. was in fact an abbreviation of "Carl".
   p. 577, "In 1917 dental researchers added to the turmoil created by the focal infection theory [when they] ... advised that no medicament sealed in an infected tooth would sterilize the tooth."
   They derogatorily note (p. 577) "Rosenow and his sponsoring institution, the Mayo Clinic, both maintained that once a tooth became infected it always remained infected." [As per Selzer in Cohen and Burns, the position of Rosenow has in fact been confirmed by modern techniques.]
   "... However ... Root canal therapy began to turn from heroic instrumentation and medication, to a more careful examination of the biologic principles. ...
   p. 579, "By 1953, many new antibiotics ... had been rushed into use... . It was found, however, that chemotherapeutic means did not completely eliminate all bacteria within the root canal. [and] ... the importance of thorough cleaning of the pulp chamber was reemphasized."

HOLMAN'S LEGACY PERPETUATED: Chase 1980
   It is frightening but nonetheless amusing, having examined the historical record and seen that the case against focal infection is fraudulent or otherwise non-existent, to see how pop medical writers have such great fun putting it down. In defense of the likes of Chase, he does base his case on Beeson's irresponsible Bi-Centennial piece; but Chase is nonetheless guilty of putting out false information.
   1980 Chase, p. 423- "The surgical and medical craze for removing what were (mistakenly) labeled as the foci of infections in people with gonorrhea and many other diseases, from arthritis to sore arms, was not the work of a scientific crackpot but two of the most honored and responsible men in American medicine and medical bacteriology, Frank Billings (1854-1932) and Edward C. Rosenow (1875- ?)". [Billings graduated from Northwestern University Medical School in 1881, taught and was Dean at Northwestern

University and University of Chicago Medical Schools, and served as President of the A.M.A., 1902].

HOLMAN'S LEGACY PERPETUATED: POP MED SPREADS IT Chase 80
   Chase 80 - asserts that the "focal infection concept was proven to be totally without foundation in 1940...", citing Beeson, 1976.

DIS-HONEST DIFFERENCES OF OPINION Grossman 1981
   Grossman 1981, p. 139, "For many years the bacteriologist ... found evidence of microorganisms in most cases when pulpless teeth were cultured by him, [while the pathologist] seldom found such evidence upon microscopic examination. These honest differences of opinion ... were reconciled some years ago. ...
   Thus did Grossman 1981 seek to elevate his misguided opinions to the level of honesty and to degrade Rosenow's scientific proof to the level of opinion. [See APPENDIX C, para. C and APPENDIX F for further discussion of Grossman 1981]

HOLMAN'S LEGACY PERPETUATED: GOING FOR THE GOLD Ingle 1985
   Ingle 1985 - p. 1, draws on Grossman 1976 for his brief derogatory references to the focal infection theory. Applauding the recent advances in techniques and instruments for root canal therapy he states: "All in all, the next decade should prove exciting and profitable for the profession and patients alike."
   Ingle et al. 1985, p. 1 refers to L.I. Grossman as the "dean of American endodontists", and refers to dentistry and endodontics as "set back by the wide acceptance of the theory of focal infection. ... The professions were not to recover their senses until well after WW II."
   Ingle et al. 1985 basically leaves it to Grossman to dispose of the focal infection theory, referring to and summarizing the latter's "Bicentennial Review" (*JAMA* 1978).
   Ingle's specialty it would appear lies in the technical areas, as evidenced in his (early) publications. For example, p. 52, among references listed are: Ingle JI and Levine M, "The need for uniformity of endodontic instruments, equipment, and filling materials.", *Transactions of the Second International Congress on Endodontics*, Edited by LI Grossman, Phila. 1958, p. 133-143; and Ingle JI, "A standardized endodontic technique utilizing newly designed instruments and filling materials", *Oral Surg.* 14:83, Jan. 1961.
   p. 560, Ingle et al. 1985: "It is now held that distant site infections may well emanate from acute oral infections via bacteriemia. An example would be bacterial endocarditis. On the other hand, it hardly seems plausible that chronic lesions cause arthritis, nephritis, etc. as once thought.
   "One must be aware, however, that certain dental manipulations - periodontal scaling or tooth extraction - might well cause a transient bacteriemia dangerous to some patients."

EYE DISEASE AS CAUSED BY PERIAPICAL DISEASE Morse 1987

AUTOIMMUNITY RECONCILED WITH "FOCAL DISEASE" Morse 1987
   Morse 1987, p. 378
   "Infectious endocarditis ... is the only definitely authenticated
example of focal disease from an oral microbial focus of infection.
   "Eye, ear and nasal infections can occur as a result of direct
extension of severe periapical phosis and conceivably can occur as
a result of hematogenous spread of microbes or their products.
Extensive investigations [Morse 1977] have been conducted of eye
conditions that apparently were related to oral foci of infection.
 Therefore if a patient has periapical disease with concomitant
eye, ear or nasal disorders, there is a possibility of focal
disease. ...
   Although it has never been proved, oral microbes (e.g., alpha-
hemolytic streptococci) may sensitize tissues at a secondary site,
such as joint tissues. The sensitized tissue antigens may then
evoke an autoimmune-type response, and a secondary disease could
result. ... A similar autoimmune mechanism has been proposed for
the development of rheumatic fever. In spite of the fact that the
concept of focal disease is not currently popular, secondary
disease from an oral focus can occur."

HOLMAN'S LEGACY PERPETUATED: ENDODONT EMPEROR Grossman 1988
   Grossman, Oliet and Del Rio, 1988 perpetuates and
institutionalizes Grossman's deplorable half-century reliance on
Holman and the inverted pyramid of ignorance devolving from it.
The authors don't specifically refer to Holman, but rather base
their confident rejection of opposition on a number of writers
referred to herein - Coolidge, Blayney, Burket and Appleton, all of
whom, as discussed above, are heavily dependent on Holman for
rejection of Rosenow and focal infection. [See APPENDIX F -
GROSSMAN FILE, for further discussion].

"CONSERVATIVE ENDODONTICS" QUESTIONED BY EXPERT Seltzer 1988
   Samuel Seltzer, *Endodontology, Biologic Considerations in
Endodontic Practice*, 2nd ed., Lea and Febiger, Phila., 1988,
briefly notes historical criticism of endodontic therapy "because
of the possible relationship of the pulpless tooth to focal
infection.", simply stating that "The certain elimination of this
possible focus of infection by conservative endodontic procedures
has been questioned.", and then proceeds to discuss possibility of
bacteremia from endodontic procedures, and vice versa. End
discussion.
   As noted above in Chapter <6>, Seltzer himself in the previous
year [in Cohen and Burns, 1987] seems to have prominently conceded
that treated root canals were found by modern methods to be
commonly infected, and that "The emphasis on obtaining negative
cultures began to be dissipated". So it would appear that Seltzer
himself seemed to be questioning the value of so-called
"conservative endodontic procedures".

HOLMAN'S LEGACY PERPETUATED Wiene 1989
RELATIONSHIP: PERIAPICAL & SYSTEMIC DISEASE Wiene 1989

p. 1, "Billings and Rosenow applied Hunter's views to the pulpless tooth, and their animal experiments indicated a definite relationship between periapical and systemic disease. ...

"Not desiring criticism from physicians and happy to take the easier way out that tooth removal afforded, dentists subscribed to wanton extraction in preference to endodontic or periodontic therapy. ...

"Fortunately some pioneer endodontists - Coolidge, Prins, Sharp, Blayney, Appleton, and others - launched a counterattack against the extractionists. ...

"By the late 1930s the corner had been turned in endodontics, and the treatment of the pulpless tooth had become an integral part of dentistry. ... The American Association of Endodontists was formed to disseminate interest and develop increased skill in the area. Under the direction of Dr. Louis Grossman of Philadelphia, international conferences on endodontics were held where interested persons from all over the world met and discussed mutual problems."

p. 25: "... almost every dental procedure ... causes some degree of bacteremia ..." (Notably, Sharp who had concluded his historical review with a quote from McNevin, also pointed out that almost every dental procedure causes some degree of bacteriemia.)

Wiene cites 3 Grossman articles from the 1960s.

PERPETUATION OF FRAUD Harty 1990

Harty, F.J., *Endodontics in Clinical Practice*, Third Edition, Wright, Condon, Butterworth and Co., 1990, notes that "treating the pulp of the tooth in order to preserve the tooth itself is a relatively modern development ... ". Mentions Hunter 1911 as having "blamed bridgework for several diseases of unknown aetiology ... It is interesting to note that he did not condemn root therapy itself but rather the ill-fitting bridgework and the sepsis that surrounded it. [Here, Harty's tertiary interpretation of Hunter, through Johnson and Grossman, takes us a step further from Hunter's clear reference to diseased tooth roots.]

"About this time bacteriology became established and the findings of bacteriologists added fuel to the fire of Hunter's condemnations. ... Whilst the theory of focal infection was not enunciated by Billings until 1918, Hunter's condemnations started a reaction to root canal therapy and the wholesale removal of both non-vital and perfectly healthy teeth began."

It is noted that here the author is clearly borrowing from Grossman, i.e., repeating Grossman's references to bacteriologists having added "fuel to the fire ...", and allegations of wholesale removal of healthy teeth [e.g., see discussion of Grossman 1976 in APPENDIX C, para. C(1)].

Proceeding to his discussion of "modern endodontics,", Harty leads with "The re-emergence of endodontics as a respectable branch of dental science began with the work of Okell and Elliot in 1935 and of Fish and MacLean in 1936." [i.e., perpetuating the lame assertions of Grossman that these two flimsy pieces justify wiping out consideration of all prior (and future) work in opposition to root canal "therapy".]

... "Gradually, the concept that a 'dead' tooth, i.e., a tooth without a pulp, was not necessarily infected began to be accepted."

Harty makes a single reference to Billings 1918, and none to Mayo, Rosenow, etc. It is particularly clear, with Harty's work, how the flawed Grossman position has become accepted verbatim as the standard.

CONTINUING PROBLEMS WITH ROOT CANAL TREATMENTS Harty 1990
HOORAY FOR HARTY FOR HIS "WORD OF CAUTION" Harty 1990

Harty concedes that attempts to formulate root filling points that would give the perfect apical seal have failed: "Unfortunately this ideal has not been achieved to date. ... [and further that] "All drugs that kill bacteria are also toxic to living tissue (Seltzer, 1988) and it is to be hoped that practitioners will realize this and abandon the use of harmful drugs for irrigation and medication of the root canal.", and "In spite of the fact that we do not know the biological modus operandi of [calcium hydroxide], it is now used in many situations. ... A word of caution is required for, to my knowledge, there are no long-term studies ..."

NEW-AGE HYPE OR ACTUAL BREAKTHROUGH? Bio-Probe Brochure 1996

There have been throughout the sordid history of root canal "therapy", a succession of claimed safer and better root canal fillings. One of the most recent, highly hyped options for use in "endodontics" is calcium oxide, marketed in the U.S. as Biocalex by Bio-Probe, Inc.

In their promotional literature, Bio-Probe duly warns of the danger of infected dentinal tubules and related problems with devitalized teeth, noting that the same disease functions occurring within the central pulp chamber also occur within the dental tubules (each tooth contains approximately 1.5 million tubules.) Although "root canal therapy attempts to completely obliterate and fill the main pulp chamber and canals ... it is impossible to fill the millions of microscopic tubules." These organisms are able to change and produce various toxic chemicals that are harmful to specific organs or systems. "This phenomenon was confirmed in a recent 1987 study by Tronstad and associates demonstrating that anaerobic bacteria ... were able to survive and maintain an infectious disease in periapical lesions of non-vital teeth. In a 1991 followup study of endodontically treated teeth, these authors recovered microorganisms from periapical lesions of all examined teeth."

Having so ably pointed out the hazards of root-canal treated teeth, Bio-Probe than asserts that this involves only ten percent of root-filled teeth; claims their product will expand, fill and seal the root canal and dentinal tubules; and recommends their product be used to treat root canals if not used as the "final ... therapy". Bio-Probe estimates that 30 million root canals will be filled annually by the year 2000. This is probably correct or perhaps even an understatement.

However, there is much in the Bio-Probe piece that is not correct or misleading. Primarily it is fundamentally flawed in that it comprises a rationalization as to why teeth can be saved, rather than an objective view of whether this is possible. The entire slant is that it is desirable and feasible to save teeth, that other methods were/are deficient, and that their product overcomes all such objections. In contrast, the record seems to clearly indicate that <u>all</u> devitalized teeth are infected, all previous efforts at root fillings have failed, and as Harty has noted above, there are no long term studies with the Bio-Probe produce (or even proper short term ones, i.e., studies using Rosenow's methods.]

Bio-Probe attributes "much of the current confusion in the minds of the public about the efficacy of root canal therapy" to Dr. George Meinig's book "Root Canal Cover-up". Bio-Probe then segues into how "establishment" dentistry gives a much different picture, but nonetheless how establishment methods are deficient, suggesting that Bio-Probe's product can resolve the situation.

Bio-Probe's first, and only "Endodontics" text, citation, is Ingle's 1994 text, which as discussed above in the "Con Chron", parrots the mortally tainted works of Grossman.

On the basis of the foregoing, positions of both Bio-Probe and its affiliate Foundation for Toxic-Free Dentistry must be challenged due to their ultimate reliance on the faulty, fraudulent legacy of Holman and the unavoidable conflict of interest between the commitment to saving teeth and the question as to whether this can be safely accomplished.

ENDODONTICS TODAY - BOOM OR EPIDEMIC? Walton et al. 1996

Walton, R.E. and Torabinejad, M., *Principles and Practice of Endodontics*, 2nd Ed., W. B. Saunders Co., Phila., Pa, 1996, notes that "There are not enough endodontists to perform all the endodontic procedures needed by the public. Undergraduate students who elect general practice must be trained to treat uncomplicated cases." No mention is made of the problem of focal infection, except that prophylactic antibiotics are discussed for medically compromised dental patients.

Part II: *Dentistry, Deception, Quackery*

APPENDIX F: THE GROSSMAN FILE

   INTRODUCTION: GEORGE MEINIG, DDS, REMEMBERS LOUIS GROSSMAN

   George Meinig, D.D.S., a now-retired dentist living in Ojai California, was a founding member of the American Association of Endodontists more than a half-century ago, and was honored at the fiftieth anniversary of that organization. Meinig has recently published a book entitled *Root Canal Cover-up*. While Meinig asserts that the facts concerning hazards of oral foci, including pulpless teeth, were downplayed by a particularly vocal sector of the dental community, he acknowledges that he is not aware of an actual conspiracy, nor does he accuse Grossman or any other specific individual of participating in such a conspiracy, except to credit the works of Percy Howe and John Buckley, in particular, with having undermined the works of Weston Price.
   Meinig relates that Howe reported on attempts to repeat Price's experiments using normal mouth bacteria, and consequently and understandably failed. Buckley, supposedly a friend of Price's, reportedly expressed confidence in the bacteriological work of Price, Rosenow and Haden, but rejected their conclusions regarding pulpless teeth; he did not see how infected teeth which seemed to show excellent bone repair after root canal therapy could still be infected, noted that some patients did not improve after devitalized teeth were removed, and challenged the validity of attributing improvement, when it did occur, to tooth removal.
   When asked about Louis Grossman, Dr. Meinig remembers him as a very intelligent man. If indeed that is true, and we have no reason to assume it is not, then a good case may be made for crediting Grossman's intellect in part with the infliction of numerous diseases, suffering, and early demise of millions of people over the last half-century, certainly more deaths than caused by all the armies of all the world's wars during that period - and the needless killing continues.
   Meinig relates that the main and continuing argument of endodontics advocates against Rosenow's work, which has frustrated opposition to the practice, is the accusation that Rosenow injected large doses of bacteria into laboratory animals, and that is why they became ill. This argument was bogus when it was first raised before 1920, insofar as all the laboratory animals injected by Rosenow in his early experiments had received uniformly sized (albeit large) injections, and the bacteria respectively located in the animals' organs that corresponded to the diseases in the human hosts. Thus the objection over the size of injections was at the outset simply nonsensical, a "red herring", just plain irrelevant.
   Nonetheless, in 1919 and 1921 Rosenow discussed the specific objection of large doses, and showed how the same qualitative result was obtained with small doses. Furthermore, all of Rosenow's work after 1920 was performed from the perspective of

sensitivity to the issue of large injections. So how can it be
that the "red herring" of large doses has persisted into modern
endodontics mentality?

In response to Dr. Meinig's having highlighted the issue of
dosage as critical in the historical mix, the writer reviewed his
notes and found that Grossman's authoritative 1976 Bi-Centennial
review of focal infection question had emphatically rejected
Rosensow's works based on this issue. This led to a review of the
works of Grossman, in order to better assess his role in
perpetuation of Holman's fraud and associated subversion of facts
concerning focal infection.

OBSERVATIONS ON THE WORKS OF LOUIS I. GROSSMAN (12/06/01-3/24/88)

Holman alone is not the entire story. Yes, the essential core of
literature advocating root-canal "therapy" by numerous writers,
from the 1930's through the 1950s and even up to the present, is
indeed incestuously and unanimously dependent on Holman's fraud as
the foundation of opposition to Rosenow. But among these opponents
one name stands out particularly - Lewis I. Grossman.
From 1940 through the late 1980s, Grossman came to be regarded as
root-canal "therapy's most prominent advocate, and must be given
much of the credit for the popularity of root-canal treatment in
modern times. In the process, Holman's fraud and derivative
articles provided Grossman with a comfortable base on which to
build, but Grossman went far beyond. The record shows that he was
able to build up the field of endodontics, and secure his long-
lived prominence within that field, through a careful and
consistent policy of ignoring, arrogantly ridiculing or otherwise
essentially misrepresenting the wealth of information that proves
that root canal "therapy" is clearly not therapeutic. Modern day
practitioners, confidently resting on Grossman's construct, have
all but eliminated reference to historical controversy over the
safety of root-canal "therapy".
As the generally recognized "dean of American endodontists"
[Ingle 1985], Louis I. Grossman aggressively promoted endodontics
throughout the world with international conferences, under the
sponsorship of the American Association of Endodontists. In
fairness to Grossman, he may not have been fully aware of the
manner in which the pivotal Holman work had fraudulently
misrepresented Rosenow. Like his cohorts, he initially seized upon
the Holman conclusion as evidence supporting the validity of root-
canal therapy, in opposition to those who maintained pulpless teeth
were invariably infected and served as foci, or "nests", from which
organisms emanated and caused systemic diseases.
On the other hand, Grossman's own protracted, seemingly
despicable behavior even makes Holman's elaborate, carefully
crafted deception seem somewhat elegant by comparison. And the
endodontics fad Grossman encouraged may turn out to be the major
single factor behind the likes of: the dramatic rise in incidence
of cancer over the past quarter-century, the prominence of heart

disease in causing human mortality, and many other disease conditions that continue to plague humankind.

It seems a bit unfair to expose the life's work of a now-deceased alleged "man of science" - particularly one so loved and respected by his colleagues as Louis I. Grossman, who is no longer around to defend himself - as far more detrimental than merely worthless. So let us try to keep an open mind, as we review:
   (A) his career as discussed in a "Special Issue" of the Journal of Endodontics; and
   (B) his published works.

A. "A TRIBUTE TO LOUIS I. GROSSMAN", *J. Endodontics*, (Jan. 82, Vol. 8)
   The following several discussions relate to items in this issue.
        (1) Introductory comment by editor.
        (2) Grossman's dog and monkey experiments
        (3) Book Review - Grossman 1981
        (4) Grossman: Philadelphia Root Canal Study Club, 1939
        (5) Grossman: Birth of American Association of Endodontists
        (6) Grossman's 1940 textbook excerpt
        (7) Grossman's impact: 11 editions, 6 languages, 48 years.

(1) Louis I. Grossman <u>was</u> endodontics.
   "His was the impetus that initiated, formulated, and implemented the multifaceted events that were essential in the recognition and maturation of endodontics. Simply stated, endodontics, as we know it today, would not have existed were it not for Louis I. Grossman. ..." Irving J. Naidorf, Editor.

(2) Grossman's experiments regarding pulpless teeth; v. Rosenow:
   The experiments of Rosenow, and others validating his views on this subject, will fill several volumes when assembled in one place, and involved thousands of animal experiments using consistent and continually-evolving and improving methods. Add to this the independently validating works of Haden, Price, Austin and Cook, Rhoads and Dick, Swanson and Van Kirk, and many others, and we have many more thousands of experiments demonstrating that pulpless, root-filled teeth are apparently invariably infected; in contrast to vital teeth without caries or pyorrhea, which are invariably sterile. Thus it is proper to review the report of an experiment on the subject undertaken directly by L. I. Grossman, perhaps his only such direct experiment, which in any case prominently appears in the 1982 tribute issue of the Journal of Endodontics.
   Summary: The article "Origin of microorganisms in traumatized, pulpless, sound teeth" by L.I. Grossman (reprinted from the *Journal of Dental Research*, 46:551-553, 1967) reported on experiments involving forcing bacteria into the gingival sulcus of dogs and monkeys, dropping weights on their teeth, and trying to recover the

organism from tooth pulps and bloodstream of the animals. The
report features an illustration in which an upside-down dog's head
is positioned beneath a vertical rigid plastic tube, through which
weights are dropped on the dog's teeth.

The article itself does not involve the study of, or even a
single further reference to, pulpless teeth within the text of the
article. Beyond this, it was difficult (impossible) to follow the
numbers, and the conclusion summation (that an organism was
recovered from about 1/3 of the teeth) is not supported by the data
presented; it seemed to be adding "apples and oranges".

Also, It seems a bit curious that this somewhat "thin" article
was given so prominent treatment within the tribute issue, i.e., it
was the sole technical justification for root-canal treatments
presented by Grossman therein.

Discussion: The Grossman article involved placing a test
organism, "swabbed over the labial gingiva" and "forced into the
gingival sulcus", dropping a weight on the tooth, and trying to
recover the test organism from the blood or root-tip, reporting the
recovery of an organism on a total of 19 occasions from 59 teeth of
7 dogs, and from 9 of 26 teeth of 3 monkeys, where the vital pulp
was subsequently removed from the canal and cultured. The organism
was recovered from the circulation of one monkey and no dogs.

This article seeks to support the position that pulpless teeth
are sterile, and that organisms recovered from the blood or the
tooth apex or root are the result of a trauma and come from
elsewhere.

Assessment/Gut Reaction:
Since this study did not involve pulpless teeth at all, the title
seems a bit misleading.

With all due respect, the article looks a bit like someone's
high-school science club experiment, complete with drawing of cute
dog and "Rube-Goldberg"-esque clamp device perched above it for
dropping weights on its teeth. The dog sure was cute, but his ears
seemed to defy gravity - perhaps a reflex reaction to having
weights dropped on its teeth, or maybe it didn't want to hear the
sound of impact.

It is difficult to follow the numbers and reporting; e.g., the
author states the organism was isolated a total of 19 times from
the 59 dog-teeth (of 7 dogs), but does not state how many teeth
were involved; some yielded bacterial growth on multiple (four or
more) occasions - all totaling 19 - which would mean that a smaller
number than 19 dog teeth yielded organisms. Further, it is not
clear how many of the 7 dogs had teeth that yielded organisms -
perhaps 3. Comparable data for the monkeys is not presented - only
that organisms were recovered from 9 of 16 monkey teeth. Thus, the
summary statement, that the organism was recovered in approximately
a third of the teeth, is not consistent with the data in the
article. In any case, the article doesn't say anything at all
about pulpless teeth.

For this effort we would give him a "D", grading him up from an
"F" for his imagination and the cute puppy.

[It seems proper to note that Grossman's perspective in this

article is consistent with the two historical articles from the
1930s that he had repeatedly cited as evidence showing that
pulpless teeth are not infected - - neither of those articles had
involved pulpless teeth either! (See APPENDIX D - THE STERILITY
NON-ISSUE, on the flakiness of Fish article.) Nor did any of these
three instances employ the culture methods of Rosenow; whereas, as
seen in Grossman 1932 below, Grossman had long been well aware of
Rosenow's methodology.

(3) Book Review (p. S34) of L. Grossman's Endodontic Practice, ed.
10, by Abel Moreinis, notes that "The 1940 edition devotes an
entire chapter to that [focal infection] theory, attempting to
justify the use of endodontic procedures. The current edition, in
a brief allusion that acknowledges 'there was a time when the
treatment of pulpless teeth was questioned,' manifests no such
defensiveness, rather it emphasizes the evidence that in the
presence of most systemic conditions, endodontics is actually the
preferred treatment." ...
  "... In spite of my biological orientation, I am pleased to find
a book which does not overwhelm the reader with page after page of
microphotographs of the cells of the dental pulp or the effects of
various materials on the pulp. ... it is easily accessible
elsewhere ... ."

(4) History of the Philadelphia Root Canal Study Club: 1939 by
L.I. Grossman (p. S41), relates how in 1939 in Philadelphia, "... a
group of dentists made the effort to break away from the focal
infection theory, which virtually banned root-canal treatment ..."
 This Philadelphia Root Canal Study Club, according to L. Grossman,
was the forerunner of the American Association of Endodontists.
Its expressed purpose was to "study problems connected with root
canal therapy and ... to help others in practicing this important
phase of dentistry more adequately."
  "I was the founder and secretary of that study club. ..."
  Grossman refers to "the 100 percenters (those who believed that
all pulp-involved or pulpless teeth should be extracted)", with the
implication that this was some irresponsible gang of tooth-
sacrificers.
  The article concludes with a testimonial by an associate to
Grossman's "untiring efforts in gaining the recognition of
endodontics as a respected specialty in the modern practice of
dentistry."

(5) "The American Association of Endodontists: its birth in 1943",
L.I. Grossman, S43.
  Herein Grossman states "certain events developed in the late
1930s and early 1940s that led to a milieu in dentistry in which a
national organization devoted to root canal treatment could be
born." Grossman refers to a 1938 JADA editorial by C. N. Johnson
which opposed the extraction of pulpless teeth as "a turning point
away from extraction of teeth"; and to a 1940 article by Austin. A
brief review of these two articles may be of interest.

(a) The Johnson article:

    [As for Grossman's reference to this as a "turning point", it might be better described as a "turning off" point. Therein Johnson begins, admirably enough, with:]

"Heaven forbid that this profession of ours should ever arrogate to itself an undue importance. ... The moment that smugness begins to raise its foolish head, hope of advancement is irrevocably lost.

    [But then ...]

"So much for one side of the picture. Now for the obverse side. We are frequently regaled by our detractors, not only from the outside, but also by members of our profession ... ." Johnson dismisses the views of presumably-ignorant medical men who have advocated the extraction of pulpless teeth, in contrast to dentists "who had been studying the teeth for nearly a century ..."

Johnson concludes that "The one great lesson to be learned from our detractors is to ignore them."

And ignore them is exactly what Grossman did - for some 50 years. The Austin article may serve as an unfortunately-not-isolated example of the manner in which Grossman did this.

(b) The Austin article. Of it, Grossman states:

"Even that former stronghold of the 100 percenters who advocated extraction of pulpless teeth for the amelioration of systemic conditions, the Mayo Clinic, began to relent when Austin, (quoting Willus, a cardiologist at the clinic) said, 'I can, I believe safely state that in our present concept, the problem virtually narrows itself down to subacute endocarditis.'"

This little clip is grossly misleading, and does not speak well of Grossman's motives nor of his actions. The Austin article, from which Grossman extracted this truncated, out-of-context statement is actually an overwhelming endorsement of the focal infection concept by many Mayo experts in many different areas. The article included enthusiastic endorsements by experts in several fields, including gastro-enterology, lower digestive tract, ophthalmology and genito-urinary tract, e.g.:

    G.B. Eusterman, Gastro-Enterology: "... I think that the clinical, experimental and pathologic evidence is sufficient to say that foci of infection in the mouth, particularly periapical infection, can give rise to the following conditions: gastric submucosal hemorrhage and hemorrhagic erosion ..., acute [and] subacute ulcers of the stomach and duodenum", and several other related disorders. ... "I don't see how any conscientious practitioner or specialist, in the light of present knowledge, can ignore the importance of dental infection in the presence of disorders or disease of the upper part of the digestive tract. If he assumes any other attitude, I feel that he is doing an injustice to his patients and to medicine in general."

J.A. Bargen, regarding the lower portion of the digestive tract: "There are a number of conditions of the intestinal tract that are related to dental infection. Foremost among these, probably, is the streptococcal type of ulcerative colitis. Here, the relationship has been clearly shown

experimentally and clinically. Removal of periapical
infection and perhaps even removal of pulpless teeth are of
great importance in many cases. ..."
Austin noted that "Dental infection is of considerable
interest to the ophthalmologist." As per W.L. Benedict:
"Extraction of affected teeth does not always have beneficial
results; but it should be remembered, in this connection, that
possibly all sources of organisms responsible for the eye
affection were not eradicated with the extraction of the
teeth, that organs other than the eye have been invaded and
become secondary foci for the production of the same strain of
organism, or that, even after extraction, a septic pocket may
have remained in the diseased jawbone. Recurrent iritis,
keratitis, uveitis and transient disturbances of ocular
motility occur from these secondary foci after the removal of
infected teeth and are to be combated by the use of autogenous
vaccines. Some forms of eye disease that formerly were
believed to be due to autotoxemia, injury, blood disease or
rheumatism or were idiopathic have been demonstrated to be due
to the actual presence of bacteria carried to the eye from
suppurative foci about the teeth or tonsils. ... Attacks of
eye disease from dental sepsis may be of any degree of
severity."
G.J. Thompson: "The relationship of infections in the genito-
urinary tract to focal infection elsewhere in the body,
particularly infected teeth, is definite. On several
occasions, I have seen acute prostatitis, pyelonephritis,
acute cystitis, etc., develop subsequently to the extraction
of the infected tooth. Such infections seem an acute
manifestation of a previously existing chronic infection, and
the acute flare-up is undoubtedly evidence of the
relationship. Chronic infections of the prostate, bladder and
kidney will often not respond to therapy until dental foci
have been eliminated. ... Any effort that dentists make to
call these facts to the attention of the general practitioner
and to the urologist is very worth while."
Austin himself, in the Section on Dental Surgery, concludes
with the recommendation, "if the patient's physical condition
is such that all suspected foci should be eliminated", to
remove not only "teeth that are grossly involved both
roentgenographically and clinically" but also to remove "teeth
that are pulpless, but otherwise roentgenographically normal,
and teeth that are well-restored, comfortable and serving
their useful purpose." In other words, Austin concluded that
even these teeth are to be considered "suspected foci" and are
to be removed. (In an earlier 1929 study, this same Austin
[and Cook] had shown that virtually all pulpless teeth, x-ray
negative as well as x-ray positive, are infected, and
virtually all normal vital teeth are not. (See Chapter <6>,
Table 4.)
Willus, the heart specialist, was clearly an exception within the
Austin article, as compared to Austin's own and the predominant

view at Mayo, when he stated "Regarding the question of dental sepsis and disease of the heart, I can, I believe, safely state that, in our present concept, this problem virtually narrows itself down to subacute bacterial endocarditis. ... There are now numerous instances in the literature wherein subacute bacterial endocarditis has followed the extraction of an infected tooth. ... So far as the other forms of heart disease are concerned, no tangible evidence exists at this time clinically linking dental infection with cardiac disease." [It is noted that a number of recent articles (circa 1990s) have discussed evidence of such links.]

Not only did Grossman ignore the predominant pro-focal-infection tone of Austin's article, but his ambiguous wording surrounding the truncated Willus quote suggested an interpretation of the Austin position that was diametrically opposite to its actuality. Even without Grossman's erroneous implied suggestion, the question may be raised as to whether his selective ignoration may in any case be considered a form of deception. As such, this seems not to reflect favorably on the long and very public career of L.I. Grossman, which seemingly is characterized by a tendency to employ such methods.

[Grossman goes on to list the founding members of the association, which included George W. Meinig of Evanston, author of the recent book *Root Canal Cover-up*, and who remembers Grossman in a favorable light. (See MEINIG REMEMBERS GROSSMAN below). Grossman was appointed to the Advisory Committee, the constitution committee, and the group in charge of the scientific program.]

(6)   An excerpt posted from Grossman's 1940 textbook provides another example of misrepresentation in support of the preferred endodontics-advocacy position, this involving the work of William Hunter at the beginning of the century. In his 1940 edition, Grossman asserted that Hunter only criticized crowns and bridgework, and not pulpless teeth, basing this on a "much overlooked but very important editorial in the JADA [22, 659, 1935]. In fact Hunter did refer to diseased tooth roots as causal focal infective locations - the editorial was wrong, and Grossman perpetuated the error in his textbooks for a half-century, from 1940 through 1988! Perhaps Grossman (for 50 years), Sharp in 1937, and Harty in 1990 were all unaware of the actual statements of Hunter regarding "tooth roots". Either way, perpetuation of this gross error does not reflect well on any of them.

Grossman 1940 goes on to assert that "the recovery of bacteria from pulpless teeth does not per se indicate that infection is present. Only when the presence of microorganisms produces a reaction - inflammation, at least - can infection be said to exist." As shown by Rosenow, Price and Haden, etc., symptomless infections are the worst type, insofar as the bacteria nave ready access to the bloodstream and hence do not "back up" and cause a reaction and inflammation.

Grossman 1940 attempts to equate the focal infection concept with fads in medicine. It is ironic that root-canal therapy turns out to be the most harmful fad in history.

Grossman 1940 criticizes Rosenow for a technic which "devastates" the laboratory animal and produces lesions in every organ, an argument Grossman would continue to raise for decades. Whereas, this argument was partly an irrelevant "red herring" and otherwise incorrect, but it continues to be thrown up against Rosenow even now thanks to Grossman's persistent reference. (See APPENDIX C, Para. C(1).)

(7)   The broad and continuing scope of Grossman's hoax is seen in the publication of eleven editions of his textbook, first called Root Canal Therapy and as of 1960 called Endodontic Practice, over the period 1940-1988, and translated into Spanish, Portuguese, German, Italian, and Japanese. In all, Grossman's textbook may have killed more persons around the world than that other famous American export, guns.

(8)   Institutionalization of Holman's fraud: It is noted that as of 1982 the Journal of Endodontics' Editorial Board of 13 included Ralph Bellizzi, and the Scientific Advisory Panel of 18 included Samuel Seltzer and Franklin S. Weine. As seen in Figure 1., these three authors' (as well as Grossman's) works in point of fact have served to perpetuate the Holman legacy (of fraud), dependent as they are (concerning the justification for root-canal therapy) on articles which directly enshrine Holman, "hook, line and sinker". The clear implication is that Holman's fraud is deeply and integrally implanted in the field.

B.   A REVIEW OF SOME RELEVANT PUBLICATIONS BY L. I. GROSSMAN

Grossman 1932 (J Dent Res XII, 595) describes apiscotomy, a method to obtain cultures from periapical tissue, and an improved type of instrument to perform these procedures.

Grossman 1932, J. Dental Research, XII, 939-44, in his early work reported on the use of Rosenow's glucose-brain broth to determine the status of periapical tissue after root-canal therapy. Most findings were negative, but there is not sufficient information to determine if method was or was not deficient.

Grossman 1938, JADA 25, May, 774-6, discusses bacteriologic examination of pulpless teeth, noting that "of 150 teeth cultured just prior to filling, 58 percent were found sterile. In the 42 per cent, bacteria were still present, and had the dentists filled the teeth, the entire purpose of root-canal therapy would have been defeated." [this writer's emphasis] Grossman states "Hormone broth, Rosenow's glucose-brain broth, Rosenow's liver broth or Holman's broth is a satisfactory culture medium." ... "Generally speaking, three successive positive cultures should condemn the tooth as a poor risk, in which further root-canal treatment would be unwarranted." It is further noted that the tubes are only slightly filled with fluid, in contrast to Rosenow's requirement of deep tubes.

Grossman 1940, 1946
- is wholly dependent on Holman and derivative articles for
rejection of Rosenow position, referring specifically and
prominently to Holman's fraudulent and otherwise insupportable
purported refutation of Rosenow's concept of elective localization.

Grossman 1946:
    States: "The specificity of the bacteria involved has not been
proved and the evidence favoring the theory of elective
localization is so open to misinterpretation and so limited in its
practical application that it cannot be considered as a help in the
solution of the problem. A certain general bacterial adaption to
environment is accepted by everyone, but factors on the side of the
host are more variable and far more important."
    Grossman 1946, p. 156, labels as a "misconception ... that Hunter
(1910) aimed his shaft of criticism against the pulpless tooth",
asserting that Hunter's target was "the accumulation of filth
around ill-fitting crowns and bridge-work." Technically, "weasel-
wordedly", the Grossman statement may be correct, in that Hunter
did not specifically refer to "pulpless" teeth.
    Whereas, as reported in the 1911 *Dental Register*, 65, p. 579-96,
William Hunter in his section on "Oral Sepsis", clearly refers to
diseased tooth roots on which dental work is built (p. 589): "Gold
fillings, crowns and bridges, fixed dentures, built on and about
diseased tooth roots form a veritable mausoleum over a mass of
sepsis to which there is no parallel in the whole realm of medicine
and surgery." Hunter illustrates the dangers of diseased tooth
roots in three specific instances (pp. 592-6). Just how Hunter's
work could be interpreted as excluding pulpless teeth can only be
attributed to a form of semantics bordering on mysticism.
    Grossman 1946, p. 158, suggests that "The recovery of bacteria
from pulpless teeth does not per se indicate that infection is
present. Only when the presence of microorganisms produces a
reaction - inflammation, at least - can infection be said to
exist." [Whereas Rosenow and others have proven this false.]
    Grossman 1946 [as in 1940], p. 159, sought to pick apart a 1917
Rosenow article [Dental Cosmos 59, 85], ignoring the succeeding 3-
decades' work of Rosenow and others which confirmed these early
findings again and again.
    [Particularly notable is the exclusion of Rosenow's responses to
criticisms over the years, particularly responses to Holman's 1928
article and Reimann and Havens' 1940 article. For example, no
mention is made of Rosenow's 1940 contribution to the Dental
Centenary Celebration, sponsored by the American Dental Association
and Maryland State Dental Association, which had specifically
covered all points in the Reimann and Havens article.]
    Rather, Grossman 1946, p. 159, refers to the conclusion of
MacNevin and Vaughn: "In a most comprehensive review of the
literature, MacNevin and Vaughn analyzed the evidence for and
against focal infection and concluded that the proof submitted by

Price, Rosenow and others, has its limitations from the standpoint of both technic and interpretation of results."

   Grossman 1946, p. 160, quotes Holman on elective localization and also cites Reimann and Havens.

   Grossman 1946, p. 162, cites Slocumb et al., who "concluded that foci of infection were found to be a factor only in 'an occasional case of coronary thrombosis or acute pericarditis' ... [Slocumb's *JAMA* article was overall in fact an enthusiastic endorsement and confirmation of Rosenow's work; Grossman extracted and mentioned only the reserved and atypical comment of a cardiologist discussed by Slocumb] ... and on the basis of a study by Binger and Woods they felt that a closer relationship exists between glomerulonephritis and foci of infection since, in 21 of 65 cases reported, improvement followed removal of tonsils or mastoid infection. No mention was made of dental foci of infection in these cases."

   p. 165-6: "The most indicting evidence against the pulpless tooth has without doubt come from the bacteriologic laboratory. Grossman cites "the two outstanding investigations [Grossman deemed] particularly valuable" because they involved different methods and yielded essentially the same results. One study involving 429 teeth examined in situ obtained growth from 72% of pulpless teeth v. 43% of vital teeth; and of 1500 extracted teeth, growth was obtained from 87% of pulpless teeth and 55% of vital teeth.

   [This last is Haden's reported result. We are reminded that Haden had attributed such differences, pulpless v. vital, to experimental error, with the fact of the difference considered to be still conclusive.]

   Grossman 1946 asserts, p. 166, that if it be taken into account that when organisms are recovered from root surfaces of teeth, that "infection is not necessarily implied, thereby the bacteriologic evidence against the pulpless tooth is not so damning." [Here Grossman discounts Rosenow's and others' safeguards against accidental contamination.]

GROSSMAN IGNORES ROSENOW METHOD Grossman 1960

   Grossman 60 [*Oral Surgery* ..., September 1960, 1131] published a bacteriology study, purportedly an "Evaluation of a method to determine the presence of a focus of infection" (O.S., O.M. and O.P., September 1960, 1131.

Grossman 1960
- in discussing "Endodontic treatment of pulpless teeth" (JADA 61, 1960, 671-6, notes that "67 percent of pulpless teeth studied were found to be infected". "The need for culturing root canals in pulpless teeth is even more urgent than in vital teeth". Grossman noted that "pulpless teeth are more commonly infected" than vital teeth.
- used brain heart infusion broth, not dextrose-brain broth..
- also notes that "the bone, as well as the root canal, may serve as a temporary nidus for microorganisms. If endodontic treatment has as its objective the elimination of microorganisms from teeth

with infected root canals, then culturing of the canals is the touchstone which determines whether that objective has been attained." (Commendations to Grossman for this, and a call for acknowledgment that it can never be attained.)

Grossman 1976
- - refers to "controlled" clinical and laboratory studies which supposedly refuted position that root-filled teeth are infected, but gives no references except his own earlier articles, which all lead back to Holman.
- - ridicules Rosenow's early (pre-1919) animal experiments based on large doses, ignoring Rosenow's having specifically addressed this point in 1919 and 1921, and ignores all of Rosenow's work from 1919 to 1958.
   Thus, more than a half century after the non-issue of large injections had been first addressed by Rosenow and averted in his subsequent four decades of work, Grossman continued to ride it as a key objection to Rosenow's work - simply because he had nothing else to work with. (See also APPENDIX C, Para. C.)

HUNTER GAVE DENTISTRY BLACK EYE Grossman 1976
   Grossman 1976, p. 83, referring to the third 50-year period in the history of endodontics in the U.S., p. 84, "The focal infection theory promulgated by William Hunter in 1910 gave dentistry in general, and root canal treatment in particular, a black eye from which it didn't recover for about 30 years. ...

FOCUS OF INFECTION CONCEPT TRACED TO PARREIDT 1889 Grossman 1976
   "In 1889, Parreidt in his book *A Compendium of Dentistry*, wrote 'According to recent observations, it is possible, in case there is a focus of suppuration in any portion of the body, for the microorganisms to pass from this into the blood, and thence they may find lodgement in any part of the body, when the conditions happen to be suitable for their development.' Almost every disease from arthritis to zoacanthosis was believed to be caused by such foci as infected teeth, tonsils, and prostate gland." Hunter's address was printed in *Current Literature*, a popular outlet, and publicized further in newspapers.

GROSSMAN SIMPLY INCORRECT Grossman 1976, p. 84
   "Many articles of a post hoc, ergo propter hoc logic appeared in medical and dental literature purporting to show that because a tooth was removed and the patient recovered from an illness - including blindness - all pulpless teeth should be removed. When controlled studies - of both a laboratory and a clinical nature - were made, there was little left to defend the focal infection theory." [Grossman gives no references, and asserts these unsupported, insupportable and false assertions as fact; note Grossman in 1988 continues to cite the authoritative bacteriologic studies of Haden 1928, which studies overwhelmingly supported Rosenow and the concepts of focal infection and elective localization.]

p. 86, "The focal infection theory, that created dissention among dentists, and between dentists and physicians, was destined to die a slow, reluctant death, leaving many people edentulous. The leaders of the dental profession challenged focal infection and defended root canal treatment in the 1930s."

Grossman 1976 refers to the editor of *Dental Cosmos* Edward C. Kirk, who in 1930 said "We are not yet fully awakened from the nightmare of ruthless tooth destruction which has shaken the very foundation of dental practice."

Grossman 1976 asserts that (quote?) "The focal infection theory was still fighting for its life in the 1940s, but its death knell was sounded by controlled clinical studies by members of the medical profession at a number of research institutions in this country." [We may refer to Grossman's earlier works, which make clear that his only foundation in this statement is the Holman/Reimann & Havens conglomerate, i.e. there is no foundation to it.]

Grossman 1976, p. 87: "The 1940s were marked by the renaissance of endodontic treatment. The focal infection theory no longer influenced the medical and dental professions and was all but forgotten. ... [It is offered that the concept of focal infection will be remembered long after Grossman has been forgotten, except as an opponent of truth and misguided agent of death.] ... In 1943 a small group of dentists interested in endodontics met in Chicago to form the American Association of Endodontists."

GROSSMAN'S FISHY CONTAMINATION ARGUMENT   Grossman 1981

It is noted that from 1940 through 1988, Grossman sought to discredit all work accomplished prior to 1936, including all of Rosenow's work, alleging contamination. Grossman based this charge on two articles, one in 1935 (Okell and Elliot) and one in 1936 (Fish and MacLean), neither of which by the way involved the study of pulpless teeth.

These flimsy pieces were apparently all that Grossman could find that he could offer up against the incredible, irrefutable, monumental works of Rosenow, which exposed Grossman's prior five decades of work as a sham, waste, and atrocious danger. Further, regarding the specific question of contamination as discussed by Reimann and Havens in 1940, Rosenow showed that large differences in results with vital v. non-vital teeth could not be simply attributed to contamination.

As might have occurred with the Holman fraud, the Fish and MacLean article would likely have been long-forgotten and properly ignored as at best insignificant, had Grossman not repeatedly referred to it as having been so significant. It's true significance is that aside from the Holman fraud, it is apparently just about all that Grossman was able to muster, in 50 years of trying, in support of his faulty position advocating the retention of pulpless teeth. For that reason, Fish and MacLean 1936 has already been given far more space here than it otherwise substantively deserves (see APPENDIX D above).

Grossman 1988
- misrepresents Hunter as having not referred to tooth roots.
- misrepresents Haden as "probably" having used aerobic methods, whereas these (from 1928) and Rosenow's (from 1914) had always involved oxygen gradients.
- prominently cites Haden's authoritative bacteriologic work, without reference to the fact that Haden implicated roentgenically negative teeth as being equally as damaging as roentgenically positive, and called for all infected teeth to be extracted.
- refers to the "interest of the investigator" as a factor in results, implying that Rosenow's work was deficient, whereas this incredibly hypocritical statement in fact aptly described Grossman's own consistent mode of operation.
- avoids all reference to Rosenow, Billings, Mayo, Price and others (with the exception of Haden, whose work is not properly explained) who conclusively confirmed that root canals are hazardous.

Grossman 1988: As in Grossman 1940, the authors refer to Hunter's "historic 1910 address in Montreal in which he condemned the 'golden traps of sepsis,' the ill-fitting crowns and bridgework of his day" and how this "inexplicably" resulted in an attack on the devitalized teeth. "Within twenty-five years, nearly 2000 papers on focal infection were published, many concerned with oral focal infection. During this period, a few voices were raised to stem the hysterical tide and to return endodontic care to its proper role in the healing arts."

This edition came out in the year of Grossman's death, so it seems clear that this and other misinformation from previous editions had by then been duly passed on to his successors.

Thus, as in Grossman's earlier work since 1940, the claim is made that two articles in 1935-6 invalidated the extensive works of Rosenow, Haden, etc. -- an article by Okell and Elliot, and one by Fish and MacLean, to overshadow the extensive works of Rosenow, etc.

(Please see commentaries above in Grossman 1981, Fish and MacLean 1936, and Okell and Elliot 1935).

"Appleton maintained that the function of root canal therapy is to render the canal and periapical tissues sterile." [If this continues to be the function, then, as per Seltzer 1987, it's a flop; i.e. it does not perform this function. (see Chap. <6>).

Grossman et. al. 1988's expression of wonderment at how Hunter's work was "inexplicably" extended to devitalized teeth simply ignores Hunter's specific reference to "diseased tooth roots" and the proofs of Rosenow in this regard. Is it possible that his younger co-authors had not bothered to read the Hunter work directly? Apparently so.

Truly inexplicable is why Grossman refers to Haden at all, in that Haden's work is an articulate, persuasive and irrefutable endorsement of Rosenow's work and the principles of elective localization and focal infection. While Grossman also refers to Haden's work as relates to fundamental oral bacteriology, his reference to it as probably involving aerobic bacteria seems a clear indication that Grossman was either unfamiliar with or chose to misrepresent Haden's work, which had long been concerned with reduced oxygen gradients. And of course, Grossman makes no mention of the Haden assertion that "a large percentage of [pulpless teeth] are in fact infected" and are "apt to be a focus of systemic disease".

Grossman 1988, p. 234, aptly highlights the importance of the subjective factor in works examining the bacterial flora of the root canal, referring to the "interest of the investigator." [MIRROR MIRROR]

Grossman 1988, p. 235, acknowledges the existence in root canals of "probably fastidious or obligate anaerobes requiring special conditions and media to survive and to grow."

p. 238, Addressing the problem of culturing these organisms, Grossman correctly states "tall tubes, filled to a high level, should be used for culturing in preference to short tubes, to provide different degrees of oxygen tension at different levels in the culture medium." However, no attempt is made by Grossman to relate this to his discussions of Haden's work, which work had in fact used such methods, nor to Rosenow's insistence on this point.

Overall, from 1940 through 1988, Grossman:

- - asserted or implied Hunter did not indict diseased tooth roots, which in fact he did.
- - referred prominently to Haden's 1928 bacteriologic work, without reference to the fact that it strongly argued against the practice of root-canal therapy.
- - asserted or implied that work supporting the concept of focal infection, and the associated implication of root-filled teeth, had not been confirmed or was otherwise deficient; whereas several workers, particularly Haden, had confirmed Rosenow's work.
- - ignored and avoided reference to any of Rosenow's work after 1917 (i.e. through 1958!), and did not refer at all to him in 1981 and 1988.
- - declared all studies prior to 1936 invalid due to contamination, based on Okell and Elliot, 1935, and Fish and MacLean 1936 (neither of which involved comparisons of pulpless teeth v. vital teeth; see APPENDIX C, para. C (2) "WEAK CONTAMINATION ARGUMENT ...", above).
- - served as an authoritative citation for generations of endodontists, e.g., Crowley 1946, Topazian 1960, Wolfson, Easlick 1951/1953, Burket 1971, Harty 1990, etc.

In 1992, in "A personal remembrance of Dr. Louis I. Grossman", *General Dentistry*, March-April 1992, 141-2, Lawrence I. Shepard relates about Grossman, who died 24 March 1988, that the writing style of the time when he worked with Grossman involved an "entertaining side" which "included wit, pitches for proprietaries, and some personal attacks" and that Grossman "never stopped using his witty personal writing and lecturing styles."

APPENDIX G: J.A.D.A. CHRONOLOGY - THE EARLY YEARS

J.A.D.A., July 1922, Vol. 9, No.7
   In Editorial "Radicalism Gone Mad", JADA Editor Otto U. King notes that "during recent years ... altogether too many teeth have been extracted through a distorted point of view as to the significance of focal infection, and the relation of the teeth thereto. While the profession needed a stirring up on the role which the teeth may play in disease, yet the extreme to which the extraction of teeth has been carried is not creditable to dentistry." King suggests "a large element among dentists have been stampeded out of their judgment and ... influenced to extract many teeth which should have been preserved."
   Beyond and "in line with the craze for extracting teeth", King asserts that "the so-called 'surgical removal of teeth' has been carried beyond the bounds of reason ... . To curette all areas from which teeth have been extracted - even diseased teeth - is a radical procedure which is not justified."

   [Inserting here, for want of a better location, the comments of G.V. Black seven years prior. Black was the unquestioned top dental authority in the early 20th century. Following are his comments on this subject, which are very much in agreement with emerging awareness of the hazards of residual bone infections:
   Black, G.V., *Special Dental Pathology*, 1915, 388, "chronic Osteitis of the Maxillae":
   p. 388 - "Chronic osteitis may be defined as death of bone, cell by cell. ... It is a condition of inflammation and disintegration which is progressive in its character, involving the bone in absorption and separation of its parts, in which we have a soft mass that may enclose more or less small hard particles of necrosed bone.
   "The condition of the progress is such that the bone is disintegrated cell by cell., instead of being destroyed en masse as in necrosis. Chronic osteitis shows a very decided disposition to continuous slow progress, attacking and softening the bone to which it makes approach, often hollowing out the cancellous portions of large areas of bony tissue. ... The disease is generally marked by what we would term a chronic condition in its whole progress.
   p. 389 - "It is a rather curious fact that chronic osteitis seldom occurs in the lower jaw, and most frequently in the incisor region in the upper jaw. ...
   p. 389 - "symptoms. There is practically no pain and very slight, if any swelling in cases of chronic osteitis. the temperature will seldom exceed one degree above normal. The subjective symptoms are so slight that cases will often run for years without the patient being conscious of anything wrong. ...
   p. 390 - "Whenever there is uncertainty as to the extent of the affected area, a radiograph should be taken. One will occasionally be surprised by the radiograph that the condition has involved much more bone than was expected and may have denuded parts of the roots of several teeth."

p. 390 - "Treatment. The treatment of chronic osteitis is
surgical, and should be radical. The area should be opened freely,
and every particle of the softened bone removed until good, sound
bone forms all of the walls of the cavity. This removal is
accomplished usually and for the most part by spoon-shaped
curettes, or large burs in the engine. Then the cavity should be
irrigated to remove the debris.

"Generally when all of the softened bone is removed, the case
makes a good recovery. ... When several teeth were involved, I have
generally extracted them."

J.A.D.A., October 1922
HEROES OF THE EARLY A.D.A. - THOMAS B. HARTZELL
High on the list of A.D.A. all-stars is former ADA president
Thomas B. Hartzell. In particular we must address his work, with
Henrici, which indicates that the invasion of the tooth root is a
long drawn out process, and the question as to whether any sort of
caries is not to be equated with the inevitable demise of the
tooth. (See APPENDIX D, above.) Additionally, some earlier
articles of Hartzell are worthy of note, e.g. the following three
from 1916: "The mouth as a factor in the pathogenesis of heart,
kidney, and joint inflammations." *Jour.-Lancet*, xxxvi, p. 215-229
(1916); "Some evidences of the importance of the dental path as a
source of serious localized and general infections." *Jour. Nat.
Dental Assn.*, iii, p. 172-185; and (with A.T. Henrici) "The dental
path; its importance as an avenue to infection." *Surg., Gynec. and
Obst.*, xxii, p. 18-27.
Hartzell served as President of the ADA in 1922, while Otto King
was secretary, and in an October 1922 article, "TEN YEARS TO LIFE",
addressed some aspects of the problem of oral focal infection. For
example, p. 831-2, he stated that dentistry has "helped to produce
the evidence that secondary anemias ... [are] dependent upon
infectious bacteria growing, for the most part, in the mouth and
upon the teeth."
Further, he asserted that "in our enthusiasm to save the teeth
themselves, we have sometimes lost sight of the greater thought
that teeth are only a part of the human mechanism concerned in the
digestion and assimilation of food and that they are subject to
infectious processes rendering them a menace to the life of the
individual even though they are playing their mechanical part in
the nutritional process. This oversight I concede to be the
greatest error into which our profession has ever fallen."

J.A.D.A., November 1922, p. 981
An article by A.C. Potter, "Why the Present-Day Reaction against
Tooth Extraction", asserts that "The dental profession of today is
face to face with one of the most important subjects any group of
men has ever had to face, namely, the subject of focal infection.
... ... there is no more harmful toxin than that from the
streptococcus group. ... Think what it means to have these toxins
circulating in the blood day in and day out, for in many cases,

years. ...

"Modern dentistry of the past few decades is largely responsible for its occurrence in the mouth. But in view of our ignorance on the subject in the past, this is entirely excusable. However, in view of our present knowledge there is no excuse for its continuance. ..."

Potter refers to "the almost ever present article decrying and condemning useless tooth extraction". Potter suggests that physicians "were perfectly justified" in wonderful expectations to come from such extractions, but that this was merely "the prelude, the introduction to a vast amount of research that was to follow. Potter called for improved examinations which might result in elimination of other foci of infection, other than the teeth, prior to tooth removal, with specific mention of tonsils and sinuses, as well as heart, gall bladder and prostate gland. (It is noted that Rosenow referred to these as secondary infections, with possible exception of tonsils, but advocated removal of teeth first; as does Potter, Rosenow suggested the mere fact of tooth removal may be insufficient due to the presence of secondary infections in other locations; in such situations, Rosenow secondarily advocated the use of autogenous vaccines, and where possible the removal of secondary foci, e.g. tonsils, etc. Potter does not mention vaccine, but rather suggests the removal of other foci before the teeth. It is not clear how this might be done, particular in 1922, particularly in such a case as when the secondary focus is the heart.)

Potter's comments on tonsils and bone infections seem to warrant repeating:

"The tonsils" I do not think that the man lives who can tell an infected tonsil by looking at it. It must be manipulated and pressed hard. One is often rewarded by pus from an innocent looking tonsil. The tonsil that is most frequently condemned - the hypertrophic tonsil - is really the least offensive. The small submerged tonsil with gaping crypts is the real offender." ...

On the subject of bone infections, "the second great cause of the failure of tooth extraction is due to poor radiograms, impossible of correct interpretation, and to unrecognized areas of alveolar osteomyelitis occurring in the edentulous areas.

"These osteomyelitic areas are diffuse, non-limited and the possibility of absorption and secondary systemic involvement is infinitely greater than from any other lesion found in the mouth. These areas are exceedingly vascular, the capillaries traversing the infectious material like a net-work, differing markedly from the familiar granuloma where the capillaries are peripheral traversing the connective tissue wall only. Radiographically these osteomyelitic areas appear as diffuse areas of increased radiolucence, in which the characteristic irregular appearance of a normally regenerated socket is absent, the shadow being usually quite dark and of even density. A description of the operative procedure for the removal of these foci is not within the province of this paper.

Jan. 1923, Vol. 10, No. 1
  In the editorial, "What of 1923?", Editor King states "We
seriously hope that in the coming twelve months there will be fewer
good serviceable and normal teeth extracted "on suspicion," than
have been sacrificed during the year just past.

February 1923, Vol. 10, No. 2
  Herein is provided a report on the activity of the Research
Commission by Chairman Frank O. Hetrick, followed by an editorial
by editor Otto King relating that although the Research Institute
had closed, research was continuing under the auspices of the
A.D.A., as discussed by Hetrick. King seeks to emphasize how in
the past research had involved too great a personal sacrifice on
the part of individuals, whereas the current plan involved grants
to institutions independently involved in research, with associated
economies. King did not specifically refer to Price, but the
implication seems clear that King was trying to rationalize the
closing of the Institute with the suggestion that the ends of
research were being better served with the current plan.
  In Hetrick's report we find some discussion of current efforts,
plus details relating to the closing of the Research Institute,
including a report by Price.
  On-going research detailed by Hetrick included work directed by:
- T.B. Hartzell at U. of Minnesota on bacterial growth, starch
digestion, TB serum test, and Bright's disease;
- Percy Howe at the Forsyth Infirmary on caries and pyorrhea;
- A.D. Black at Northwestern U. on treated apices, permeability of
dentin and cementum, and toothpastes, etc.;
- Guy S. Millberry, Chicago College of Dental Surgery on apices in
partially filled roots;
- Henry C. Ferris at the U. of California on saliva and pathology;
- A.D. Black at the Dental Index Bureau on a classified index to
the literature.

  Hetrick's report included an accounting by Weston Price on "the
activities, financial and otherwise of the Institute since its
closing in 1920. In accordance with the resolution adopted at the
annual meeting of the Corporation in July, 1920, the work was
terminated. ..." The remainder of Price's report is concerned with
financial matters.
  Hetrick concluded: "Too much credit cannot be given Weston A.
Price for the grand work that he did in building up this department
of our professional activities, and that his name may be known as
the moving spirit in our early struggles, the Research Commission
has taken the following action:
  "Resolved: That after all obligations are paid upon the Research
Institute of Cleveland, that the funds received from the leasing of
the property, shall be known as the Weston A. Price Research
Commission Fund. All honor to this grand man. We believe that
better work is being done in our department each year and we most
earnestly hope that we may see no backward steps in the years to
come."

July 1923, Vol. 10, No. 7
   The editorial "The Need of Balance" notes that "Very frequently a
new idea runs away with its advocate, and leads him to do things
which are not only ridiculous, but which are actually harmful." In
this editorial, King particularly criticizes "so-called 'surgical
removal of teeth'".

   John P. Buckley is pictured as A.D.A. President. It is noted
that Buckley, along with Percy Howe below, were particularly
singled out by George Meinig, D.D.S., in *Root Canal Cover-up* as
having been instrumental in the anti-focal-infection movement.
   Weston Price is pictured as Chairman of the Histology, Research
Section.

Sept. 1924, Vol. 11, No. 9
   C.N. Johnson is pictured as "President Elect".

Jan. 1925
   C.N. Johnson writes lead editorial ("What is Research?") as
"President", at the invitation of the editor.
   In the succeeding months Johnson, as president, continues to
appear on the editorial page, and officially becomes editor in
December.

April 1925
   Johnson emphasizes the "real force in numbers", extolling members
to recruit their fellow dentists into the A.D.A. "Forty thousand
members banded together in an enthusiastic endeavor to elevate
dentistry could put it on a plane never dreamed of by the men of
even a decade ago."

June 1925, Vol. 12, No. 6
   In this issue's lead article, entitled "FADS AND THEIR EFFECTS",
A.D.A. President C.N. Johnson recounts some of the deleterious
practices that have caught the fancy of dentistry. These include:
 - "the fad of filing teeth for the purposes of creating what were
erroneously called self-cleansing spaces ... [accomplished by]
grinding away the tooth so as to leave large V-shaped apertures
looking toward the lingual surface ... . this fad took a strong
hold on the profession. Nothing but the bitter experience of its
victims stopped the fad, and brought the practitioners to their
senses.
 - "the so-called 'New Departure Creed' [advocating the use of
guttapercha in the place of gold foil] ... in the late seventies
and early eighties ... created a real furor in the profession. ...
[This] fad of plastics threatened to sweep gold foil from our list
of filling materials."
 - other fads discussed were hypnotism, cataphoresis, copper
amalgam, analgesia for cavity preparation, administering gas for
the filling of teeth (resulting in "an unfortunate crop of dead
pulps"), and the use of emetin for treating pyorrhea. Of this last

Johnson notes "we can only blush for the extent to which this remedy was forced on a helpless public. The fact that it was all done with the best intentions goes only a short way toward ameliorating the embarrassment with which we must recall this period of our practice. It is well that a merciful public forgets and forgives. ... ."

Johnson then moves to more recent times and fads which to his way of thinking "have a more sinister aspect". He includes in this category the surgical removal of teeth and the condemnation of pulpless teeth.

Some observations:

Both of these practices interrelate, as discussed below, and had been championed by Weston Price and others. A fact seldom mentioned by opponents of "surgical extraction" is that the particularly forceful impetus for removing residually infected bone came from the unquestioned leader in dentistry in the early 20th century, G.V. Black. Advocacy of this necessary work is receiving renewed and proper interest, aided by improved radiographic technic which confirms the continued presence of residual bone infections caused by the retention of, and following removal of, pulpless teeth; Johnson, in somewhat typical, subjectively abusive fashion, suggests that the motivation is "for revenue only",

Ironically, the practice most strongly defended by Johnson, retention of pulpless teeth, will certainly come to be known as the most harmful fad in the history of health, whereas he takes the opposite, totally backwards and incorrect view - that the <u>removal</u> of these permanent nests of infection is "one of the outstanding and disastrous fads of the century in medical and dental practice."

In that Johnson himself has introduced the profit motive as a factor, it is safe and fair to suggest that, albeit probably unconsciously, Johnson is blinded by the inherent conflict of interest that characterizes dentistry and renders it incapable of taking a truly objective stance on the question of the proper disposition of pulpless teeth. If appreciably carious, or even slightly carious, teeth and all root-involved teeth must be extracted, this appreciably cuts back (to just about nil) on the allowable level of tooth mechanics - carpentry, filling, crowning and sculpting, etc; in other words there would thankfully no longer be much (of this in-any-case harmful) activity for the dentist to perform, except, one might think, for extractions. Think again.

The ill-advised practice of retention of pulpless and otherwise diseased teeth, in terms of insidious residual bone infections, mandates surgical extraction and removal of associated infected bone. Thus, there would appear to be enough work to keep all dentists, with some supplementary training, working overtime to correct the deplorable situation dentistry has wrought. Of course, this is difficult work, so not all dentists would be able to move into it. At the same time, there would in any case seemingly be an increased demand for the jeweler-type skills that are demanded by modern dentistry - - related to the manufacture and fitting of proper prosthetic devices ("choppers").

Johnson on the pulpless tooth (continued):
Addressing "the present attitude of some men toward the pulpless tooth, I unqualifiedly term it a fad and a delirium ... a species of professional insanity ... ." Johnson suggests that if the pulpless tooth is damaging, it is due to the power of suggestion:
"The pulpless tooth has been a prolific medium for frightening many people into a state of hysteria over the condition of their health. ... If a person is not feeling quite up to the mark ... [and] is told that a pulpless tooth in his mouth is pouring out poison in his system, it is not long before he can actually feel that poison coursing rampantly through his veins. ...
"I freely, frankly and humbly admit that I am not a research worker in a pathologic laboratory, but I have had a somewhat extended clinical experience ... . And I am thoroughly convinced that, in our present prejudice against pulpless teeth, we have gone far astray, and I hereby make the strongest possible plea for a return to conservatism and sanity. ... my present prediction is that we shall arrive at the truth more surely be careful clinical observation and study than through the medium of laboratory research. ..."
This is a theme to which Johnson will return - that research is no substitute for clinical experience. Accordingly he has closed his mind from the outset to that which Rosenow and others so elegantly have proved - that these insidious oral focal infections, particularly including root-filled teeth, relate to and cause long-term chronic illnesses. Rosenow, Price and others were actually able to cause these same diseases in laboratory animals, using organisms from pulpless teeth or pulpless teeth themselves, thereby fulfilling Koch's postulates. Thus those who have subverted proper consideration of Rosenow and Price, etc., have not only subverted those works but also the tradition of Koch and Henle, and of medical progress in general. All this in order to save -- teeth? Yes, because that is the only way they could, and even today's dentists can, continue practicing their craft as currently defined.
 And this must cease, as it is the only way we can, and must, save our lives.

August 1925
In an article, "THE PULPLESS TOOTH FROM A BACTERIOLOGIC AND EXPERIMENTAL STANDPOINT", Russell L. Haden, M.D. notes at the outset that very little experimental proof concerning the causal relation of a focus to a disease in individual cases is available except that of Rosenow and co-workers and of Price. I have attempted by cultures of dental infection and by certain animal experiments to obtain further facts ... ."
Haden describes how he and associates followed closely the technic of Rosenow in examining some 1307 root tips, including 392 vital teeth, 490 x-ray negative pulpless teeth, and 425 x-ray positive pulpless teeth.
As seen in Table 6, below, pulpless teeth overall are several times as likely to yield 100+ colonies in deep agar tubes as vital

teeth, and far less likely to be sterile in broth. X-ray negative teeth are nearly as likely to be infected as are X-ray positive teeth.

Haden notes that "Some of the teeth considered as vital were probably pulpless since all were not tested for vitality and others had large cavities and might well have already had infected pulps.

TABLE 6. QUANTITATIVE CULTURES FROM PERIAPICAL INFECTION

Group	Number Cultured	% Showing Colonies in Deep Agar Tube, by Number Colonies			No. Sterile in Broth; Per Cent
		1+	10+	100+	
Vital	392	14	5	1	46
Pulpless	915	61	51	33	18
X-Ray Negative	490	54	44	24	
X-Ray Positive	425	70	63	44	

In the case of the pulpless teeth, Haden notes that "The incidence of infection is almost as high as in those with positive roentgenographic findings.   Infection in the tooth with negative roentgenographic findings is probably more serious from the systemic standpoint than when the findings are positive, since little resistance in the part of the body is indicated and absorption is probably more rapid. ... Several times during the past two years I have compiled statistics concerning the cultures and the percentages have remained almost constant.

"These results show that infection is actually present around the root tips ... ."

"To determine the disease-producing power of the bacteria from dental foci, we have injected rabbits with the original broth cultures recovered from the root tip. Two rabbits have been injected routinely with 5 cc each of the culture from a single tooth or with the mixed cultures from several teeth. In most instances, the animals do not die as a result of the injection."

Of his results Haden notes "The high incidence of lesions shows clearly the great disease producing power of the bacteria from chronic foci and leaves no doubt that such organisms are capable in a high degree of causing disease in man."

Haden notes that this particular data does not provide proof in individual cases of a causal relationship of dental infection to systemic disease. However, he offers that "The truth of the theory [of Rosenow that bacteria tend to localize in certain tissues] has been conclusively demonstrated by Rosenow and his co-workers. I have been able to present confirmatory results in diseases of the eye, the stomach, and the kidney, and in cases of onychia. The proof seems absolute that bacteria do have such a selective tendency. Those who have questioned the theory after experimentation have failed to observe the necessary requirements as far as oxygen tension and rapidity of work is concerned. ... The proof that, in certain cases, there is this causal relation ... is best presented by a few case histories ...". Haden presents cases involving pulpless teeth, wherein the organism taken from pulpless teeth of persons with various diseases caused similar symptoms in laboratory animals, including endocarditis, arthritis, paralysis, hyalitis, pyelonephritis, duodenal ulcer, and multiple onychia.

Haden concluded that "A very high percentage of teeth that are negative roentgenographically harbor infection. ... In selected cases, one can prove the unmistakable tendency of bacteria to from chronic foci to localize in certain parts of the body. These cases afford valuable experimental proof of a causal relation of a chronic focus to systemic disease."

It is noted that [p. 930] Haden refers to Holman: "A culture on blood-agar of the roots of the extracted tooth showed a profuse growth of Streptococcus nonhemolyticus 1 (Holman)." This organism was injected in a rabbit and replicated in the toenail an infection that had been seen in the fingernails and toenails of the patient.

During the question period following the presentation, Haden offered that contamination in the case of pulpless teeth would not likely be greater than the small percentage of positive cultures encountered in vital teeth, which might to some extent be possibly considered as reflecting contamination.

He presented evidence that 53 percent of animals injected with bacteria from patients with peptic ulcer developed the same, v. 7% of animals injected with other bacterial.

A member asked, "Isn't a 5 cc dose of pure culture an overdose for a rabbit weighing, say, 1,500 gm.?" Haden's response: "That is a very fair dose. Rosenow has used up to 75cc, but we use only 5. This is a big dose -- much more than a patient ever gets at one time, but it think it is a perfectly fair amount to use to get comparative data in the cases studied. Patients are receiving small doses over a long period of time instead of a single large dose such as is given the rabbit."

In the dialogue, Price asked a Dr. Bunting, "Do you deem it possible to sterilize infected cementum while the tooth is in the mouth?" Bunting responded, "If the cementum is extensively involved, I would either amputate or extract."

This point would be exploited a few months hence by Johnson, in what one might speculate was a trap laid for Price by his "friend" John P. Buckley, in cahoots with C.N. Johnson. This is, of course, speculation; however, it is clear that the question of sterilizing the cementum in the mouth had been raised by Price in JADA prior to his upcoming debate with Buckley, and further that Johnson and Buckley would thus have been aware of this apparent "weakness" in Price's argument.

Dec. 1925, Vol. 12, No. 12
Herein tribute is paid to the career of Otto King, former editor of JADA, King had served as General Secretary of the ADA since 1913. At that time he began publishing a bulletin which developed into the JADA, serving as its editor until Sept. 1925, when a new editor was appointed; King continued as Business Manager.

In the editorial, "The Buckley-Price Debate", newly appointed (Sept. 1925) editor C.N. Johnson casts the deciding vote in a debate between Weston A. Price and John P. Buckley, held before the Odontographic Society of Chicago, Oct. 12, 1925. This is Johnson's first official editorial as editor.

The debate resulted from a challenge from Buckley to Price, in reaction to a paper presented by Price in the previous year, and attracted an audience of 1500.

Johnson jumps into the fray due to "the transcendent importance of this question of pulpless teeth [which] makes it imperative that the widest consideration be given it from every possible source."

Johnson focuses in on "the pivotal point made repeated by Dr. Price to the effect that a pulpless tooth cannot be sterilized in the mouth, quoting a statement by Price in the "debate" that "It is practically a physical impossibility, if not completely so, to sterilize infected cementum by treating through the dentin", this due to the impervious nature of the dentinocemental boundary.

This, asserts Johnson, has the result that "Dr. Price has unconsciously been 'hoist on his own petard.' It is a poor rule that will not work both ways, and if it is impossible for the agents of *disinfection* to pass this barrier, it is equally impossible for the agents of *infection* to pass. Consequently, *the only thing necessary to make every pulpless tooth perfectly safe to the host is to seal the apical foramen*. [Johnson's italics] There is no escaping this contention -- if Dr. Price is right.

"Mayhap, Dr. Price is right, and mayhap that accounts for the well-known clinical fact that there are countless thousands of pulpless teeth being retained in the mouths of people today to their great comfort and advantage, and with not the slightest injury to their physical well-being. There is no intent, at this time, to take sides in the recent debate, but merely to refer to this point, which was so strongly emphasized by Dr. Price, and to call attention to its practical application."

Johnson dismissed the remainder of information presented with: "much of the confusion is caused by clouding the issue with too many irrelevant statistics which have no practical bearing on the main issue, and which take no account of the actual happenings in the mouths of actual people. The farther we get away from concrete clinical experience, ... the farther we shall wander from common sense and the truth ... ."

Thus did Johnson dispense with Price, and by all accounts Price pretty much seems to have abandoned further efforts to convert the ADA on the issue of pulpless teeth. (In conversations, Dr. Meinig has indicated his understanding that the subversion of the focal infection concept was pretty much beaten back in the 1920s; it seems clear that this "debate" [trap] was most likely a key event.)

A cynical mind might suggest that this debate may have been instigated by Johnson, who had followed Buckley as ADA President; presumably Price had previously referred to the impossibility of sterilizing the cementum via the dentin, and could be expected to do so again. Johnson may have been previously prepared to nail

Price, and relied on the set-up opportunity of a challenge by Buckley to "debate" to execute the planned elimination of the nasty and embarrassing problem of Weston Price.

Regardless of whether this was a set-up, Johnson's very convincing argument was clearly (1) the turning point for Price's activism within the ADA and essentially the apparent deathknell for any form of opposition to root-canal therapy within the ADA (it is noted that in any case the Research Institute had been discontinued, as per reference below by Buckley); and (2) faulty.

The situation posed by Price involved an hypothetical non-vital tooth in which infection exists both within the dentin and in the cementum. (Presumably the infection had progressed from the dentin, through the apical foramen, to the cementum, although they might conceivably have had independent origins.) Price first emphasized the near-impossibility of sterilizing even the dentin, discussing difficulties in doing so even when the dentin was removed and immersed in a disinfectant. Thus the possibility of sterilizing the dentin in place was seen as quite remote, and to then go beyond and sterilize the cementum was even further removed from the realm of the possible. Price emphasized that because of the relative impermeability of the dentinocementum boundary, the disinfectant would have to travel through the apical foramen and hence to the infected cementum. In view of the insurmountable task of sterilizing even the dentin, the prospects of sterilizing the cementum were viewed as anything but promising.

Johnson twisted this around, implying that therefore it didn't really matter if infection continued to exist within the pulpless tooth, so long as the apical foramen were sealed, since this would prevent the escape of harmful organisms into the bloodstream. Even if it were possible to seal the apical foramen, which Price's and other works have showed to not be possible, Johnson's quick fix would have no impact on an existing infection in the cementum, which was the subject of Price's discussion in the first instance. Nor would this have any therapeutic effect on the continuation and expansion of any infection into surrounding bony tissue, nor on the status of the apex and indeed the entire tooth as a "locus minoris resistiante", a location which offers no resistance to colonization by harmful blood-borne organisms. Plus we are reminded that it appears to be impossible to seal the apical foramen in any case, so that minute organisms from the non-vital root canal or miles of dentinal tubules within the tooth would in fact continue to seep through the apical foramen and into the bloodstream.

The Price position, as presented in the JADA debate, highlighted four areas: (1) that the high death rate from degenerative diseases was due in part to pulpless teeth; (2) that it is impossible to sterilize infected cementum in the mouth; (3) that susceptibility varies, therefore consideration of treatment must do likewise; and (4) new evidence from blood chemistry implicates toxic substances from infected teeth can and do disturb or destroy normal defenses and function. Numerous tables and figures were provided, illustrating Price's position. It is notable, and in sharp contrast to Buckley, that Price's presentation was void of personal attacks and/or innuendo.

WITH FRIENDS LIKE THESE...

In his presentation, following Price, Buckley sought to emphasize from the start that "If it becomes necessary for me to speak plainly and to the point in presenting my side of the question, I want the audience to know in advance that there is nothing personal intended." Buckley proceeded to assert that Price was "personally responsible for much of the criminal practice that is being done today", because of his published writings and his position as head of the Research Institute of the ADA. Buckley does credit Price "for stimulating the spirit of research in dentistry more than any other man in the profession. This in itself is sufficient justification ... for all the time and money spent by the profession in furthering the work of the former Research institute." Buckley emphasizes the importance of the truth and keeping an open mind to the facts. He proposes to show that "normal tissues of the body are not always germ free", and that limitations of the roentgenogram, as discussed by Price, might be repeated regarding bacteriologic findings. He blames the publications of Price and others for justifying "the radical stand many men are taking today with reference to the ruthless extraction or so-called surgical removal of pulpless teeth, challenging Price "to assume the responsibility for the radical extraction of all pulpless teeth" or to alternatively advise caution, dwelling on the assertion that Price has not made his position clear. Buckley accuses Price of being more concerned with saying what he thinks than thinking what he says, and further, that "he travels too rapidly or he does not stay in one place long enough for those of us who are a little sluggish to get our perspective or bearings.

Referring to animal inoculation, he notes "Rosenow is reported to have used up to 75 cc in a single dose ... Is it any wonder that the innocent young rabbit is overwhelmed?" On this subject he notes Haden uses only 5 cc. and has expressed the need for caution in interpreting results of animal experiments, admonishing Price for not having issued like precautions. While he recognizes Rosenow as a bacteriologist of note, he criticizes him for a lack of special work along the line of dentohistopathology.

[Thus Buckley, a former A.D.A. President, lends great weight to Grossman's and others' continuing criticism of Rosenow's having used large doses in his early animal experiments, despite the fact that this issue was a "red herring" from the start, and addressed directly in any case by Rosenow some years earlier. Further, among those cited by Buckley on the question of dental pathology, in contrast to Rosenow, are Hartzell and Henrici; but when we go to their actual work, we find them aligned with Rosenow. As discussed above, Henrici and Hartzell in 1919 showed that in most teeth with caries or pyorrhea the root has already been invaded with bacteria.]

Beyond this, Buckley attacks Price thusly: "he gives us absolutely no hope for saving a pulpless tooth under any condition.

My God, men! Whither are we drifting? There is such a thing as carrying science, so called, far beyond the realm of the ridiculous and plainly to within the limits of criminality." Of Price he asks, "does he report only such as would seem to justify his preconceived ideas? And ... does this not prove that as a scientific investigator his is either incompetent or unreliable or both? Certainly, it must be suspected that he lacks the tireless and irresistible courage of complete sincerity and sanity." Buckley concludes his barrage with "God giving me the strength, I will spend the remainder of my life, if need be, correcting this damnable and criminal practice for which you, sir, Dr. Price, whether you realize it or not, are in large measure responsible."

January 1926, Vol. 13, No. 1
   In "Editorial, 1926", Johnson calls for "a clarification of the pulpless tooth problem. This question has assumed a status where something more definite must result from its consideration, and it is hoped that the coming year will do much toward clearing up some of the present confusion concerning it."

March 1927, Vol. 14, No. 3
   In the editorial "Critics", Johnson, offers "Critics are seldom constructive. ... usually their chief aim seems to be to find fault. ... Unconsciously, the critic assumes an air of superiority which renders him oblivious to the opinions of others ... . Such a thing as humility is alien to his nature ... .
   "Through all the ages the critic has never inspired one noble impulse in a writer or painter ... . .. the greatest function in life is to be helpful, and almost the worst sin is to obstruct."

Dec. 1927, Vol. 14, No. 12
   Percy Howe is listed as President-Elect, serving as A.D.A. President in 1928-9. Howe, along with Buckley, have been prominently mentioned by George Meinig in his book, *Root Canal Cover-up*, as having been instrumental in contributing to the suppression of the works of Weston Price, etc.

June 1928, Vol. 15, No. 6
   In "The One Thing Needful", editor Johnson notes "In that perennial topic, the pulpless tooth, there is assuredly need of a better understanding and a more uniform opinion on the part of members of our profession ... . Greater sanity seems to be entering into the situation, but there is still much room for the harmonizing of theories."

Sept. 1928, Vol. 15, No. 9
   "The Swing of the Pendulum" editorial is dedicated to the question of the pulpless teeth, asserting that "The question of the pulpless tooth is still with us, but it is much nearer a solution than it has been for several years, and there is evidence of greater sanity in its consideration. ... Just why a well filled pulpless tooth should have been considered an undoubted menace, it

is difficult to understand, in the face of the clinical fact that countless numbers of such teeth have been retained in the mouths of patients for many years ... ."

Herein Johnson reprints a query and response published in JAMA May 26, 1928, on limitations of roentgen-ray diagnosis of dead teeth, effect of dead teeth on adjacent tissues and health, and modern opinion on filling root canals.

On the first point the response offers: "The roentgen ray is of no value in diagnosing teeth with dead pulps except in those cases in which infection, following the death of the pulp, has penetrated and destroyed bone about the apex of a root. The roentgen ray does not show infection of bone, but reveals an area of bone which may have been destroyed by infection or otherwise."

The response goes on to assert "There is no such thing as a dead tooth unless it has been extracted. ... A tooth from which the pulp has been removed may not present any menace to the patient. ... "There are records of many thousands of cases in pulps have been removed and root fillings made which, from all the evidence available, do not show any sign of infection after many years."

Johnson accentuates that despite its "manifold blessings", "the roentgen ray does not show an abscess, or pus, or infection of any kind", and urged that the profession and people not be made to suffer from such limitations.

Johnson proceeds to discuss the problem of pulp canals that are not filled to the apical end, and the assumption that they must be refilled, suggesting that "Nature might [fill] the empty root end, and thereby protect it.

"... now we have something to supplement clinical evidence in the form of demonstrable scientific evidence." Johnson refers here to a paper by Edgar D. Coolidge in this same issue which portrays "how unfilled spaces are sometimes closed by Nature in such a way that infection is prevented."

Acknowledging that 100 percent of pulpless teeth cannot be saved, Johnson asserts many more might be than in the past, and quotes Coolidge as having said "A comparison of roentgenograms with histologic sections shows that it is not necessary to extract all teeth with imperfectly filled root canals."

In the article referred to by Johnson, above, Edgar D. Coolidge, "Pulp Pathology and Treatment Problems", presents numerous microscopic photos which seem to show reparative processes occurring in teeth in which root-canals have been treated and filled. Some evidence of regeneration and filling in of imperfectly-filled roots is exhibited.

By all accounts Coolidge was a good scientist and honorable person, and it cannot be disputed that the information he presented is genuine. However, there is nothing in this work which would indicate that the works of Rosenow, et al.. had been superseded or rendered invalid; the subject of bacteriologic culturing is not addressed herein. The conclusion to be drawn might best be characterized by analogy to the chicken whose head is cut off and continues to run around the farmyard for a time. Despite the fact that the pulpless tooth serves as an insidious focus of infection, with its dentinal tubules teeming with organisms and the surrounding bone becoming increasingly infected (often with minute organisms which would not necessarily be evident in conventional microscopy, but which are clearly evident in more exacting photos as reproduced in George Meinig's *Root Canal Cover-up* and Weston Price's studies, etc.) it would appear that other aspects of biological function and healing elsewhere related to the tooth may continue. Indeed as we get further from any infected focus, life processes may be expected to proceed normally, except when condition are appropriate for the spread of the infection to such a location. This would help explain why a pulpless tooth would not immediately be rejected by the body, and thus explains the favorable clinical experience with retaining pulpless teeth that has encouraged dentists to retain them. But they are in fact infected, continue to be infected, and continue to contribute to systemic disease, just as proved by Rosenow et al..

At some point the beheaded chicken will stop running due to the beheading, as the night follows the day.

January 1929, Vol. 16, No. 1

Buckley, J.P., in the article "The pulpless tooth, its pathology and conservation; a new method and technic of filling root canals", offers material for emphasizing two essential points concerning the pulpless tooth and the position of the ADA. Firstly, the expressed purpose of this article, and unquestionably of the ADA with the rare exception of the likes of Weston Price and his Research Institute, has never been to determine whether it is safe to retain the pulpless tooth but rather how it may be conserved. Secondly, the continual seeking for a new method and technic of filling the root canals is clear testimony that previous methods were failures.

This continues to the present day, as seen in the critical comments of Harty 1990, a prominent contemporary endodontist. Every suggestion of a "new" method says something is wrong with the old. But it is continued and defended, with all the power of the association, until a better "new" method comes along, with its revolutionary promise to improve the situation. At the same time there is never an admission that the old method is deficient. What a crock - a financially-motivated, arrogant, criminal crock.

O.K. so maybe that's a bit overboard, because it may be categorically stated that virtually all practitioners truly believe they are doing the right thing. But at the same time, there is something drastically, logically very wrong here. If not criminal, there is certainly intellectual negligence at work here. And while probably no one is directly thinking that this is a financial threat, there is an unavoidable, irreconcilable conflict of interest built in.

May 1929, Vol. 16, No.5

In "This is Refreshing", the editor takes note of an editorial in the *Journal of the Indiana State Medical Assn.* for March, entitled "The Inconsistent Craze for Removal of Teeth". Johnson emphasized this was written by a physician, who refers to the "veritable slaughter of tonsils and teeth". The Indiana editorial comprises most of Johnson's *JADA* editorial, and calls for the retention of "so called dead or pulpless teeth that have been cared for properly by a dentist."

March 1930, Vol. 17, No.3
   The editorial "A New Root Filling" discusses still another "novel and even revolutionary" method for filling root canals, which "will be read with much interest by those who are concerned with the preservation of the pulpless tooth ... ". Naturally there is no discussion of the inadequacy of current or prior methods, which logic would dictate is clearly implicated by such a revolutionary pronouncement.
   The editor then goes on to emphasize the overriding importance of clinical experience to the question of pulpless teeth. "No other kind of evidence can ever take the place of clinical facts well authenticated. ... when this question of the status of the pulpless tooth is finally settled, it will be done in the clinic and the office rather than with the test tube and the microscope. ... Let us study clinical records more and resort to theorizing less."

October 1930, Vol. 17, No. 10
   In the editorial "Shall We Abandon Our Birthright?", editor Johnson gets down to the nitty-gritty of the situation, the question of whether dentistry "should sink our identity and become a specialty of medicine.
   Johnson acknowledges that "at one time dentistry begged to be taken under the wing of medicine and was curtly refused ...", asserting that "the art of dentistry has ... advanced to an infinitely greater perfection under the present plan than it could possibly could as an appendage to another calling." Further, Johnson asserts, "dentistry has never been well taught in a medical college having a dental department. ... Dentistry has not built its birthright for nothing. ... Shall all of this be swept away by the wave of a few fanatical hands? ... We shall gain little ... by the attempt at this late date to attach ourselves to the band wagon of medicine and trail behind like the little dog that has been clipped for the occasion. ... Our birthright means too much to us to go begging to any profession for affiliation. ... If we had been a failure and our policies a mistake, there might have been some logic in begging another profession to mother us... . Dentistry has developed specialties in its own field that are outstanding in their service, and it is absurd to try at this advanced stage of its growth to submerge its entire fabric in the body politic of another calling. It cannot be done."

Feb. 1931, Vol. 18, No. 2
   Editorial: "Stand Pat". "If you know you are right, stand pat."

May 1932, Vol. 19, No. 5
   Editorial: "Finding Fault." "Some writer has said, 'Nothing is

easier than finding fault; no talent, no self-denial, no brains, no
character are required to set up in the grumbling business."

July 1932, Vol. 19, No. 7
   The editorial "Cooperation between the Physician and the Dentist"
asserts "We cannot longer admit that physicians know more about the
mouth and teeth than we do ..." Johnson asserts that "Almost ever
since dentistry became a profession, there has been a constant
endeavor on the part of dentists to interest medical men in the
significance of the teeth, with very meager results ... ." But
after Hunter brought attention to the problem, "the medical
profession lost its balance and carried many of the dental
profession with them."
   Johnson asserts, in what might be termed an even evil and
certainly deliberately misleading discussion, that Hunter never
referred nor intended to refer to "focal infection coming from the
ends of pulpless teeth", but rather implies that Hunter was
exclusively concerned with sepsis from faulty or unclean crowns and
bridges, which he referred to as "gold traps of sepsis".
   Whereas, in fact, Hunter said (repeated here for proper
emphasis), "Gold fillings, gold caps, gold crowns, fixed dentures,
built in, on and around diseased tooth roots, form a veritable
mausoleum of gold over a mass of sepsis." It is clear that Hunter
did in fact refer to diseased tooth roots. Therefore it seems
clearly inaccurate, and even morally reprehensible to imply that
Hunter would have in any way excluded pulpless teeth from his
indictment. Rather the contrary seems all but certain.
   Johnson goes on to emphasize that the dentist is entitled to more
respect than the physician on the question of passing judgment on
the teeth, insofar as the dentist "has spent five years in
intensive training on this one subject ... ."

March 1933
   Newton G. Thomas is assigned as Associate Editor. He would serve
through November 1935.

January 1934, Vol. 21, No. 1
   In "Root Canals and their Therapy", Associate Editor Thomas
reviews some of the history and problems that had characterized the
field of root-canal therapy, in an atypically objective (for the
A.D.A.) assessment.
   Thomas notes that less than 20 years previous, "root canals were
of small concern. For easier opening, pulps were removed; canals
that had been open to the luck of the mouth were filled; half
pretentious attempts at sterilization were made. ..."
   On the question of sterilization, Thomas notes that while some
partially filled roots had remained negative for years, [presumably
some] "well-filled canals had developed alarming apical changes."
As a result, better operators developed, and "numerous technicians
developed who showed completely filled roots with becoming pride
... - in the films displayed.
   "then came the focal infection didactic. ... systemic

disturbances of vague origin were attributed to teeth with root tip changes. ... The market appreciation of pulpless teeth went down. The next step was that all pulpless teeth were potentially dangerous. ... What is a tooth when health is at stake? ...

"We are now in the bacteriologic era. Innocent looking teeth have been subjected to the acid test and found far from innocent. Bacteria cluster about the apices of sound, live teeth, probably owing to contamination. But the apically sound, roentgenographically good pulpless tooth has 750 times more. In other words, such a tooth keeps open house to militant germs. Resection has been suggested for feasible roots that show distress. But -- still thinking of the innocent-appearing pulpless tooth -- a resected tooth is still pulpless and welcomes its guests with the same cordiality as before.

"Still another item, but slightly considered in this connection, is root-canal form. In 1917, Hess filled canals of teeth with molten Wood's met al. under pressure. Then he removed the tooth from the cores and photographed them -- 986 of them. [see JADA Sept. and Oct. 1921.] ... The canals bifurcate, twist, skein, loop in the weirdest fashion. They show every conceivable irregularity. Marrow canals (from internal absorptive processes) run to the surface in any part of the root. Multiple termini penetrate the apex. To see them is to wonder how one could hope to sterilize them. Cleaning them is an impossibility. Filling them is out of the question. Interestingly too, no roentgenograms show more than two or three of these termini filled even when the most painstaking artist does the work. ..."

Thomas relates statements of various authorities on this dilemma, attributing to Stein, "By no means does the certainty of the know methods of root-canal treatment compare with the certainty of extraction"; Appleton, "The only practical solution to the problem of the pulpless tooth, I fear, is not to have pulpless teeth"; and Hatton, "Focal infection is no longer a theory but a principle of dental and medical practice. The solution of the pulpless tooth question is that of prevention." Thomas concludes that "Evidently pulpless teeth belong to the 'continuate and inexorable maladies,' for the time to be.

"Osler once spoke of 'maladies against which we can scarcely ever hope to have curative measures.' In that phrase, he unwittingly classed our problem as it stands. ... Caries banished, the pulpless tooth will cease to torment us."

Thomas's editorial stands out in sharp contrast to the general trend of other JADA editorials encountered during this period for its refreshing and objective perspective. Had this perspective prevailed, the situation today might well be much improved. He would contribute one additional notable editorial on the subject of pulp-involved teeth (see June 1935, below) before disappearing from the editorial pages seemingly without mention (this writer looked for, but did not see anything); whereas his assignment in 1933 had been properly noted in (see above, March 1933).

April 1935

In the editorial "A PERSISTENT MISCONCEPTION ABOUT HUNTER AND THE SUBJECT OF FOCAL INFECTION, Johnson again seeks to subvert the legacy of Hunter, asserting (as he had previously in July of 1932) that "The 'oral sepsis' of which he complains ... had nothing whatever to do with ... focal infection from the apical ends of pulpless teeth. ... Hunter never referred in the remotest way to the evils of pulpless teeth as such. He was concerned with the sepsis that came from accumulations around crowns, bridges and artificial dentures, calling them 'gold traps of sepsis.' ... he should no longer be credited with initiating the campaign against pulpless teeth, because he did not do it. ..."
Wrong. Hunter was concerned with both the sepsis and the overlying gold traps. Johnson's presentation is totally out of line and abominable. Johnson's exclusion of the fact that Hunter did refer to diseased tooth roots seems clearly diversionary and intentionally deceptive. And insofar as most practicing dentists would not have the time, or inclination, to check the facts, the power of such a diversion by a former A.D.A. President and long-time editor of the J.A.D.A. on rank and file dentistry is virtually inestimable.

June 1935, Vol. 22, No. 6
In "ROOT CANALS AND PULP", Associate Editor Thomas surveyed the history of efforts to preserve pulps, noting that G.V. Black had in 1870 reported that 38 of 42 pulps treated in 1860 had become pulpless by 1868. Black is quoted as stating "The healing power of the organ [pulp] is very low. ... If a touch is sufficient to draw blood the pulp will be destroyed." Thomas noted that in 1868, "when Witzel advocated the excision of the pulpal bulb, Black called the practice pernicious."
In 1919 Howe advocated preservation of injured pulps, offering this as the preemptive solution to the controversial problem of root-canal therapy, but Thomas characterized the foundation of Howe's optimism as frail, and further, that "The literature echoes and reechoes with the ancient thesis of small reparative power, the very early age below which success may be expected and the easy death of the pulp."
Thomas recounts Hatton's and Skillen's reports of pulpal activity after "lacerations from broaches" or other intrusions, and Skillen's report of "remaining pulp squeezed between filling and dentin wall as 'apparently normal.' To the imaginative, this held out possibilities. Evidently there are conditions in which the pulp does not die after slight hemorrhage. Under some circumstances, an abused, traumatized, tortured pulp fights for its life successfully. ..."
"At this juncture, another shadow falls across the endeavor to save pulps. We are told by Ellingham that pulps under large fillings, pulps that have become fibrotic from irritation, may be infected and infective. ..."
On the other hand Thomas asserts that "Root therapy has made tremendous progress in the treatment of accessible teeth. Such men as Hall, Blayney and Coolidge have done brilliant work in this

field. ... Says Rickert ...: 'It is now seldom necessary to extract single rooted teeth.'" But Thomas offers that "Pulp saving, to be successful, must not exclude the multiple rooted teeth." Thomas concludes on the hopeful note, regarding the problem of pulp preservation, "There must needs be failures, but it is our task to increase the number of successes and make their probability more and more certain."

Thomas continued to be listed on the editorial page masthead through November 1935, and subsequently was dropped from the listing without announcement (at least this writer didn't find one). One may surmise that his two editorials on pulp-involved teeth may have had something to do with this - the above item from June 1935 and an earlier one in January of 1934.

It is encouraging to see that Thomas was willing to take a position which was not in agreement with the powers-that-be of the time, particularly editor Johnson; but somewhat discouraging that Thomas was unable to continue and move up to the editorship when it would become vacant upon Johnson's death in 1938.

Nonetheless, for his objective perspective and courage to have it printed in the JADA (albeit perhaps when Johnson was on vacation), Newton G. Thomas is hereby awarded the first AUTOMED Weston Price Memorial HERO-IN-THE-HISTORY-OF-DENTISTRY award. Had he been able to attain position as editor of JADA, the world would probably be a much healthier place today.

June 1936, Vol. 23, No. 6
In the editorial "Laboratory Findings or Clinical Experience", Johnson once again asserts "if we cannot trust clinical evidence, we cannot trust anything." Let us pin our chief faith to the experience that comes to us through actual contact with the daily manifestations that we encounter in the mouth."

April 1937, Vol. 24, No. 4
In an editorial "Does Our Code of Ethics Mean Anything?", associate editor L.P. Anthony states "The struggle up from sheer quackery to our present enviable and encouraging status has not been an easy one." Here Anthony is railing against breaches of ethics in the form of display advertising.

In an editorial "The Changing Concept of Oral Focal Infection", Anthony offers that "the medical profession is slowly, if rather reluctantly, coming to the conclusion that the oral focal infection theory will not solve all their diagnostic difficulties ... ." Anthony notes some good has come from "this newest experience in phantom chasing", insofar as it has encouraged dentistry in "perfecting a method of treating and filling pulpless teeth ...". Anthony laments that acquiescence to the focal infection concept by dentists carries the reflection that dentistry is "largely a mechanical art, and that dental health service is based upon pseudoscience." Anthony concludes that "More serious attention must be given to the question of saving pulpless teeth, if we are to meet the obligations imposed upon the dentist by the emergencies of the passing depression."

   Here we see in advance the changing of the guard, and it becomes
ever-increasingly clear that the issue is not a small group of
dissident dentists wishing to do root canal "therapy" who subverted
the good intentions of the majority, but rather that the very
existence of dentistry and the ADA are dependent on the
continuation of root canal treatments. Price and the Research
Institute were clearly an embarrassment to the organization and its
mission; it would not have been sufficient to have merely
discontinued the work of the Research Institute, as this would have
left Price a martyr. Rather, Price had to be discredited, the
execution of which was set up by Buckley and performed by Johnson.

July 1937, Vol. 24, No. 7
   The editorial "Radicalism in Dentistry", asserts that "Dentistry
has suffered greatly through running after false gods, and the
people have often paid the penalty. ... It is easy to recall
numerous instances of failure and folly, of grief and woe following
the advocacy of certain radical and attractive methods of
practice." ...
   "When we consider the youth of dentistry as a profession, we may
well marvel at some of the evidences of its achievements. ... At
the pace we have been traveling, it is little wonder that we have
occasionally made a misstep and in the vernacular have 'come a
cropper'".

November 1937, Vol. 24, No. 11
   In "Vindication", the editor notes "we confess that we are a bit
weary of the effort that it sometimes requires to justify dentistry
to the public. ... If the teeth are intended to serve any useful
purpose in the economy of nature, the efforts to preserve them on
the part of the members of our profession are eminently justified
and essentially praiseworthy. ... The pathetic wrecks left by the
loss of the natural teeth have challenged the dental profession to
remedy this appalling disaster to humanity. ... Let us hold our
heads a bit higher, and not mope around in an implied attitude that
we are "only a dentist. ... The limit of our possibilities has not
been reached, and it never will be reached through the agency of
subserviency. We must claim our legitimate prerogative and
prestige ... ."

Feb. 1938, Vol. 25, No. 2
   The editorial, "The Beneficence of Denture Restoration", notes
"We have frantically tried to snatch the natural teeth from the
impending doom of decay and disaster, only in too many instances to
be forced back beyond the ramparts and left prone in the
humiliation of defeat. And what may not this defeat mean to a
human being!"

   In "The Broadening Scope of Dentistry", associate editor Anthony
criticizes "those who believe that dentistry should be a specialty
of medicine ... ", referring with a degree of alarm to "the

possibility of losing our autonomy if we follow blindfoldedly the
lead of those who are deceived by the dentomedical will-o'-the-
wisp."

June 1938
   In the editorial "Our Detractors", Johnson exhorts his associates
to ignore the opposition:
   "Our detractors, from certain members of the medical profession
down to the ballyhoo artists of the public press, who till recently
have dubbed us 'tooth carpenters', have done us much harm.
Fortunately, there has been of late a great change for the better.
 Medical men for the most part are cooperating loyally and happily
with us ... . The one great lesson to be learned from our
detractors is to ignore them. ... Hold up your heads, ye men of
wavering faith, our detractors are breaking ranks and the best is
yet to come."

August 1938, Vol. 25, No. 8
   Editorial page leads off with an obituary for Charles Nelson
Johnson, 1860-1938, who died on July 17. "Dr. Johnson was without
doubt the most prolific writer the dental profession has ever known
... ". This lead article closes with the notation that Johnson
"has been known for several decades as 'the most loved man in the
dental profession.'"

February 1939, Vol. 26, No. 2
   The editorial "Dentistry's Responsibility - Preparedness"
recounts how in 1840 Horace H. Hayden, Chapin A. Harris and
colleagues initiated a course of instruction in dentistry entirely
separate from medicine, which "was apparently agreeable to medicine
at that time". Anthony offers that efforts of the dental
profession, to call attention of medicine to the relation between
teeth and disease, were generally ignored until the time of Hunter,
whereupon attitudes were reversed practically overnight.
   "As a matter of fact, we were so successful in demonstrating the
fact that oral sepsis played an important role in the causation of
systemic disease, that medical thought was quickly converted to [a
state] in which too much attention was directed to mouth disease as
a cause of systemic disturbances." Thus the dentist "was forced
into a copartnership of needless tooth elimination."
   Anthony offers that "The one favorable resultant of the reaction
... was an awakening to the realization of the biological
relationship of dentistry." This in turn was reflected in a higher
grade of dentist. However, according to Anthony, "the raising of
the educational standards, with the consequent increase in time and
expense of the dental course, was proceeding too rapidly",
resulting in a reduction of the numbers of dental school entrants.

March 1939, Vol. 26, No. 3
   In "Educating the Public Dentally", editor Anthony bemoans the
"ultra-ethical restrictions that have prevented the profession
[from] the publicizing of the benefits which dentistry can render

to humanity."   Anthony offers that "this attitude ... has encouraged and frequently compelled certain classes of the public to obtain their information on dental health subjects from questionable sources."

Anthony relates that "The doubtful value of the publicity received in general was the impelling cause for the adoption of an organized method of publicity directed through the agency of the ADA. Such an agency, the Bureau of Public Relations, was established in 1931, and has since functioned as a definite activity of the ADA. As the scope of the work of the Bureau has enlarged, some two years ago the Bureau included in its activities a campaign of educational publicity through the newspapers, which ... has been particularly salutary in establishing a cooperative and wholesome attitude on the part of newspapers toward dentistry."

Anthony lauds the supplementary works of the Greater New York Bureau for Dental Information, which has even more recently served "to dispel some of the prejudices that have been unwittingly instilled in the mind of the public toward dental procedures." As an example of this work, a recent LIFE Magazine article is cited "which embodies in a wholesome manner much beneficial information on many phases of dental practice."

June 1939, Vol. 26, No. 6
A reprint of part of the first American dental periodical is presented (The American Journal of Dental Science, New York, 1839.)
Therein the publishing committee, among other particulars, stated, "The Arts of Quackery will be boldly exposed; and the public will be instructed how to avoid the impositions of ignorant pretenders."

April 1940, Vol. 27, No. 4
In the bibliographical section, Louis I. Grossman's *Root Canal Therapy* is presented, with the notations that "pulpless teeth are not being regarded as a severe menace to general health, as they were at one time." It is asserted that "although the relationship of root-filled teeth to various systemic diseases has had ample time for a thorough clinical evaluation, the exact association between the two is as faint or indefinite as ever before. ... and that the patient will be best treated by conserving as many of his teeth as is practicable. ... The book should prove useful both as a text for students and as a reference work for practitioners."

May 1940
The lead editorial, "WHY NOT SAVE THE PULP INVOLVED TOOTH?", refers to dentistry of 20 years prior having become "hysterically employed in the removal of all teeth in which the pulp was in any way involved", asserting that "this fatalistic attitude" was "almost wholly without confirmed scientific reason". "Hunter's diatribe" is characterized as having "struck a psychologically hopeful chord" to physicians who could not otherwise address many "more or less intractable conditions". The editorial offers that the passing of time and "development of much contradictory evidence" [which we now know to be non-existent), dentistry sought

"a sane and safe position" which led to the saving of teeth.

The piece repeatedly slams the opposing viewpoint, e.g., referring to "long years of trial and, unfortunately, error", "ranks of the 'hundred percenters'" being augmented by reports of "miraculous cures", and "the making of so many dental cripples", asserting that "the pulp involved tooth can be restored to usefulness ... without menace to the health of the patient ... ". The article repeatedly emphasized the conclusive testimony of clinical experience which argues for saving teeth. In this effort, asepsis is cited as the "vital principle" involved, which seems particularly interesting insofar as modern expert testimony (e.g. Samuel Seltzer) concedes that in fact that sterility within the treated root canal cannot be maintained.) It was noted that some medical internists were beginning to question the systemic-disease role of oral foci in general.

The works of Sommer and Crowley (below), in the current issue of JADA, is cited as "one of the most exhaustive and scientifically sound studies" thus far presented, "which should dissipate finally all doubt as to the ability ... to save the pulp involved tooth."

Sommer, Ralph F. and Mary Crowley, in "Bacteriologic verification of roentgenographic findings in pulp involved teeth" (cited in above editorial), from the start attack the "unwarranted sacrifice of teeth" due to misinterpreted x-rays. In rather sharp contrast to the findings of Rosenow, Haden, etc., who had demonstrated the unreliability of x-rays in that x-ray negative teeth are often in fact infected and may be worse than positive ones from the focal infection viewpoint, Sommer and Crowley in essence sought to show that even x-ray positive periapical regions were not necessarily infected and of minimal concern. They criticized Haden's exactingly careful methods as inviting contamination.

In support of their position the authors reported that "Negative cultures were obtained from all types of roentgenographic lesions. ... [and] positive cultures were obtained from teeth which appeared roentgenographically normal." It is noted, however, that their technic clearly did not conform to Rosenow's methodology, hence can in no way be considered to refute or otherwise cast doubt on the results of those who did use the proper procedure. This critical failing, coupled with the early-stated, clearly biased intent of the article, i.e., to justify the retention of pulpless teeth, at a minimum must raise questions as to whether this article indeed "should dissipate finally all doubt" as to the wisdom of saving pulp-involved teeth.

The authors reach the extreme conclusion "that there is no relationship between the roentgenographic appearance of a tooth and its bacteriologic content ... " and hence that "too much emphasis should not be placed on the roentgenogram as a diagnostic agent in condemning questionable teeth." Further, they assert that "In view of the rarity of proved cases of systemic involvement associated with teeth that appear roentgenographically and bacteriologically positive, there is considerable question as to the importance of the pulp-involved tooth as a focus of infection."

And there is nothing but sand and more sand, as far as the eye can see - to the ostrich whose head is submerged in it.

June 1941, Vol. 28, No. 6
   The editorial "SCIENTIFIC DENTAL LITERATURE?" recounts the predominance of the mechanical perspective in historical dental literature, crediting Billings and Hunter with having called attention to the relation between teeth and systemic disease and the need to broaden the dental perspective to encompass scientific considerations. It is conceded that "there will always be a certain percentage of readers who complain that scientific literature is 'over their heads,'", but that a large percentage of current dentists are in favor of scientific communications in the journal, and that "the future of dentistry ... demands the broadening of the scope of our knowledge."

July 1949
   In an article, "Dental Infection and Extraoral Disease, p. 21, Nadler, Walter H., sought to revive consideration of focal infection, presenting two case studies in which pulpless teeth were implicated as causing systemic disease (endocarditis, and iridocyclitis). Nadler concludes that the subject of focal infection continues to be important.
   In an accompanying editorial (p. 63), "Dental Foci of Infection: Good Case Histories Needed", the Nadler article and a report from the American Geriatrics Society are cited as adding "to the list of evidence favoring the elimination of all oral foci." The editorial notes that "Most physicians and dentists can cite instances in which the removal of dental infection has improved a patient's physical condition.", and expresses the hope that improved record-keeping of dental case histories "will supply scientific evidence for or against the case of oral foci of infection."

June 1950, Vol. 40,
   In "Advances in Dental Science", a major article with several contributing writers that recounts the first 50 years of the Twentieth Century, J.R. Blayney relates some details on the Research Institute of Cleveland, which had been headed by Weston Price. It opened in 1916, and was abolished in 1920 "in favor of providing grants-in-aid to dental schools or private laboratories, and fellowships ... ".
   In a sub-article, Edward Hatton refers to the "pronouncements of Hunter and Billings" due to which pulpless teeth were "black-listed", and to Price, Rosenow, and Haden, et al.., who "toured the country with their propaganda and filled the journals ... ".
   Hatton particularly cites and dwells on both Holman's "critical appraisal" and "a second thorough appraisal" by Reimann and Havens as prominently having had an impact on diminishing interest in focal infection. Thus it is seen that, by 1950, these flawed works had become ensconced in the mentality of dentistry as having largely disproved the focal infection concept. Nonetheless, Hatton notes that Irons in 1946 had reaffirmed his belief in the concept,

and Hatton concedes "there seems to be some ground for a refusal to reject radically the theory in its entirety."

   At this point this supplementary review of JADA editorials, etc. was terminated, insofar as key subsequent JADA items are already in APPENDIX E - A "CON" CHRON (e.g. see EASLICK 1951, 1953 therein.) Again, apologies for making you jump around, but it is hoped that the inclusion of this supplementary file makes it worthwhile.

APPENDIX H: POSTSCRIPT ON HOBART REIMANN

Though the writer did not encounter any sort of however-justifiable retort by Rosenow to the trickery of Holman, we do find, thanks to the kind reference of Martin Fischer (*Death and Dentistry*, 1940), a particularly notable piece of 1939 correspondence in the *Archives of Internal Medicine* responding to statements by Hobart Reimann in the same journal in the previous year. As Reimann 's 1938 47-page-long "review" may well be viewed as a preview to his shorter 1940 pivotal piece in *JAMA* (with Havens), i.e., that which was cited by Beeson in 1976 as marking the demise of the focal infection "theory", we may benefit from Rosenow's poignant remarks on this occasion on two counts: (1) exposure of the lame nature of the case against him and the concept of focal infection; and (2) the civility and solidity of Rosenow and his position. As per APPENDIX C, Para. A, above, this writer has attempted to address a number of points raised by Reimann and Havens (beyond their reliance on Holman's fraud for refutation of Rosenow's animal experiments) from the Rosenow perspective. Rosenow's comments below seem to expose anything left as malicious hot air:

"To the Editors: -- Polemics should have no place in science. I have consistently refrained from them and shall continue to refuse to try to convince by argument alone those whose views are at variance with my own. Differences founded on experiment I have considered from time to time as occasion demanded by the presentation of new or additional data and, incidental to these, have indicated so far as possible wherein lay the reason for the discrepancies.

The statements by Reimann with regard to my work on elective localization and on the use of vaccines in cases of infections of the respiratory tract are so misleading as to require consideration.[1] I can point out only (1) that from his list of diseases in which I have presented evidence indicating streptococci as the etiologic factors, he omitted four -- ulcer of the stomach and duodenum, cholecystitis and gallstones, canine encephalomyelitis and equine encephalomyelitis -- and that he neglected to state that my results have been corroborated by my associates and independently by others for most of the diseases he listed; (2) that he neglected to mention the fact that Schotmüller was the only person who really voiced disagreement with my views on elective localization at the German Congress of Internal Medicine at Wiesbaden; (3) that Schotmüller admitted in the open discussion on that occasion that the principle of elective localization was applicable in some cases; (4) that the discussion or rather presentation of confirmatory studies by many, some of whom voiced emphatic disagreement with Schotmüller's views, exceeded fourfold the allotted time for my paper, and (5) that in making rounds with Schotmüller several weeks later, an invitation I accepted at the time of the congress, I found much evidence of focal infection in his patients which had been entirely overlooked by him. Infection was actually demonstrated in 5 patients during my short visit. One had recurring attacks of cholecystitis, 2 had suffered from rheumatic fever for about two months and 2 had acute iritis. A history of an attack of acute tonsillitis shortly before the onset of the systemic disease was elicited in each of these cases, and large amounts of liquid pus were expressed from the tonsils of each by the method my colleagues and I use. Acute pulpitis with death of the pulp and draining dental sinuses occurred shortly before the attack in each of the 2 cases of acute iritis. And, finally, Schotmüller himself had been at home in bed ill with an unexplained fever for some time prior to my visit. It was clearly evident that he was an example of the very problem under discussion. His teeth were literally floating in pockets of pyorrhea, and his breath was terrible. He died several years later of cardiac failure.

In regard to Reimann 's criticism of the work which Heilman and I[2] have done on the prevention and treatment of colds and influenza, I am impelled to record the following statements: It is generally conceded, as indicated in our paper, that the initial symptoms in colds and influenza are associated with the virus and that organisms of the pneumococcus-streptococcus group are the chief cause of the subsequent symptoms, lesions, complications and death. The strains of these organisms from persons having colds or influenza possess on isolation characteristic pneumotropic virulence and other specific properties which they promptly lose on cultivation on artificial mediums. They become like the strains isolated from the throats of well persons remote from an epidemic of infections of the respiratory tract.[3] In previous work[4] the value of vaccines prepared from the freshly isolated strains of this group of organisms was demonstrated in animals and on a large scale in human beings during the pandemic of influenza of 1918 to 1920. The vaccinated patients as compared with the unvaccinated controls fared from three to twelve times better as regards the rate of attack, incidence of pneumonia, hemorrhagic edema of the lungs, empyema and encephalitis. It seems (1) that Reimann overlooked the fact that our results obtained in human beings, especially in prevention, were so overwhelmingly favorable whenever the vaccine was used as to leave no doubt of its value; (2) that the vaccine actually used for human beings protected animals against infection by streptococci regularly at hand in these diseases; (3) that he failed to consider the fact that our vaccine was prepared from strains freshly isolated in dextrose brain broth after preservation in dense suspension of glycerin (two parts) and 25 percent salt solution (one part); that vaccines prepared in this way are much less toxic and more immediately antigenic and hence more suitable for treatment than vaccines prepared directly in the usual manner from streptococci, often after almost indefinite cultivation on artificial mediums; and (4) that he seems to have missed completely the remarkable fact that a vaccine prepared in 1937 from four hundred strains of streptococci isolated during the pandemic of 1918 to 1920 and preserved in the glycerin-salt solution menstruum protected animals against the streptococcus isolated from persons ill with influenza during an epidemic in

1937. This vaccine was not used for human beings, as stated by him, but instead vaccines prepared from a number of more recently isolated strains.

Edward C. Rosenow, M.D., Rochester, Minn.

1. Reimann, H.A.: Infectious Diseases: Review of Current Literature, *Arch. Int. Med.* 62:305-352 (Aug.) 1938.

2. Rosenow, E.C. and Heilman, F.R.: Streptococcal Vaccines in the Prevention and Treatment of Respiratory Infections, *Am. J. Clin. Path.* 8:17-27 (Jan.) 1938.

3. Rosenow, E.C.: Cataphoresis as a Control of Specificity of Streptococcal Vaccines: Influenzal Streptococcus Vaccine in the Prevention and Treatment of Infections of the Respiratory Tract, *J. Immunol.* 26:401-433 (May)1934.

4. Rosenow, E.C.: Studies in Influenza and Pneumonia: IV. Further Results of Prophylactic Inoculations, *JAMA* 73:396-401 (Aug. 9) 1919.

Reprinted with permission of the American Medical Association: *Archives of Internal Medicine*, 63, 602-3 (1939), Copyright 1939, American Medical Association.

APPENDIX J: POSTSCRIPT ON W.L. HOLMAN

    Of course, we can't leave without a few final words on Holman -
his prominence; a bit more on how his attack on Rosenow was a well-
thought-out and well-executed diversion, truly a grand fraud; and
some earlier history on Holman which starts to give us an idea of
his motivations.

HOLMAN'S PROMINENCE

    In the first instance it must be acknowledged that Holman was a
well-known bacteriologist of his day. Thus we find him prominently
referred to in Haden's work, remembering that Haden was and still
is highly regarded by all parties; and in the work of Hatton, a
prominent member of the A.D.A. in the first part of the 20th
Century:

    Haden referred to Holman's Broth and Holman, in Haden 1928, p.
38: "We have found it difficult to grow many of the strains of
streptococci in the broth prepared according to Holman's
directions, so a modified brain broth has been employed. Lactose,
mannite and salicin were added to sugar-free broth in the
proportion of 1 per cent. Small pieces of calf brain were placed
in 1/2 x 4 inch test-tubes and the broth added. All strains grew
well in this medium."

    Hatton, in Black, GV, 1936 (posthumous edition, of dentistry's
"bible" as it were), refers prominently to Holman: "... the
principle of focal infection ... has advanced to a principle that
is widely used in the treatment and control of a large group of
diseases by practitioners in both medicine and dentistry, as noted
by Holman."
    Subsequent to a discussion of the early work in Ancient Assyria,
and Benjamin Rush's work in the late eighteenth and early 19th
centuries, Hatton returns to Holman: "Holman, in the article
already mentioned, names John Abernethy (1809) as another physician
who had the same notion as Rush with respect to diseased teeth."
Hatton then touches on the works of Arthur D. Black, who listed
articles from 1842 onward; Garretson's attribution of various
systemic conditions to dental disease, in 1890; W.D. Miller's 1891
use of the phrase "focus of infection" with reference to conditions
in the mouth; and G.V. Black's "antedating Miller's paper by some
seven years" with a book on the effects of toxins from bacteria in
the causation of disease.
    Grossman 1938 also referred to Holman's broth. (See APPENDIX F,
Para. B.)

A CLOSER LOOK AT HOLMAN 1928 - A REALLY ELABORATE FRAUD

    Holman 1928, pp. 68-136, begins with the sentence: "Focal
infection has changed, with increased evidence from a theory to a

principle of infection. It has often been misunderstood and misinterpreted ... ." ... In a recent letter, I have called attention to the prevalent confusion of many investigators in research and clinical medicine between the facts of focal infection and the hypothesis of elective localization as promulgated by Rosenow and his followers. ..."

Holman thus, in his fourth sentence, refers to his 1927 JAMA prelude to [this] fraud, herein executed. This 69-page article, from the outset, was a set-up to wrongfully challenge Rosenow.

Holman drops back to Mayo's reference to Hippocrates, then to Abernethy 1809, then Rush 1801-1818, Trousseau 1865 in Roethlisberger, Graves 1835 in Fischer 1920, and Winge 1869-70 in Blum 1918, as illustrative that the concept was not new.

This is followed by discussions of types and strains of streptococcus (pp. 70-75), with an offhand disregard for Rosenow's bacteriological work: "The early work by Rosenow on transmutation has little to do with the problem of today. I discussed certain phases of his work several years ago." [J. Infect. Dis. 15:293, 1914; discussion follows]

Following this Holman proposes to review literature first on various foci, then hypothesized secondary diseases, and then to return to the question of Rosenow's elective localization. Thus he discusses first tonsils (p. 76), then teeth (p. 80), then gastro-intestinal tract diseases, etc., and then other factors such as diet and vitamins, from p. 82 through p. 127, where he enters the topic of elective localization.

As he moves into consideration of Rosenow's work, Holman discusses a number of Rosenow articles, abstracting various statistics in a confusing manner, charging Rosenow with "many more instances .. . of such a confusing use of figures ... ", and insinuating impropriety with "It is impossible to evaluate the personal equation in such work ... ." p. 131-2.

This sets the stage for Holman's statement on p. 133 "I believe the proper basis on which to obtain the significance of these results is to determine the total number of animals showing a particular lesion and then to estimate the percentage of such lesions apparently induced by the so-called 'specific' and 'nonspecific' strains", and also on this page, Holman's insidious "Rearrangement of Rosenow's Results ...". This is followed soon by his conclusion on p. 135 that the hypothesis of elective localization has not been proved. The article ends on p. 136.

Insofar as Holman from the outset intended to challenge Rosenow and mounted the challenge with the fraudulent "rearrangement" near the end, it may readily be suggested that the intervening many pages were simply diversionary.

HOLMAN ON ROSENOW, 1914

Holman had been after Rosenow for a long time. In particular, back in 1914 we find him attacking the foundation of Rosenow's work on mutations, without offering any concrete contrary evidence.

In J. Infect. Dis. 15:293, 1914, "The relative longevity of
different streptococci and possible errors in the isolation and
differentiation of streptococci", Holman relates that Rosenow
claims to have effected transmutations between pneumococcus and
streptococci of various types, and proved this complete by every
known test. Holman asserts "The results of my experience and those
of numerous other workers would tend to throw doubt on many of his
interpretations." Holman asserts that Rosenow's results were due
to contamination or some other factors, and dismisses other aspects
of Rosenow's reported work with statements like " ... contrary to
the experience of all workers ...", "... I would be unwilling to
believe ... ", and "My interpretation of this ...". This brings us
to within one sentence of the "Conclusions" section, which states
Holman's conclusions, against Rosenow, without further reference to
Rosenow.

CONCLUSION, ON HOLMAN

Competition, jealousy, the possibility one's entire career was
wasted and is proven wasted due to the works of Rosenow - - that
seems to be the most logical explanation of why Holman did what he
did. Ironically, while Holman will not be remembered for his
bacteriological works, he will be remembered for his fraudulent
manipulation of Rosenow's data, and for having successfully pulled
off the most pervasive, destructive, and even grand, fraud in the
history of medicine. And we are his victims.

APPENDIX K: DENTISTRY'S LEGACY: REDEFINING QUACKERY?

   Modern dentistry is not to be confused with quackery, although there do appear to be some similarities.

   Both are falsely presented as having curative powers, both are based to some extent on fraudulent foundations, and practioners of both may well be ignorant of their respective vital flaws. And both have mercury associated with their origins.

   Nonetheless, despite these similarities, one might suggest that the main reason for not regarding dentistry as quackery is that the latter is too benign a term. "Quackery" generally denotes worthless pseudo-medical practices, often laughingly so. One thinks of snake-oil purveyors, fancily packaged placebos, arrogant pronouncers of gobbledegookism, etc. -- worthless, but harmless, except as they may cause diversion from validly beneficial actions.

   Modern dentistry is neither worthless nor harmless. Of course, dentistry does provide the benefit of extending dentition, the use of one's natural teeth for consumption of food. However, the down side is certainly worse than the sum total of all properly-considered quackery in the history of the world.

   On reflection, the very concept of dentistry is somewhat illogical. The teeth are bones, connected to the jawbone by what is basically a "joint", notwithstanding dentistry's preferred alternative terminology. When a tooth is infected, one has an ulcer of the tooth bone, an ulcer exposed to the outside elements. (Fischer characterized such infections, all tooth infections, as compound fractures.) When "decay" about this ulcer is drilled out, it is still an ulcer -- a bigger one. And when these openings are filled, the oxygen gradient is much reduced and they cannot heal; on the contrary, the reduced oxygen situation favors the growth of harmful bacteria. Reaming out the root-canal(s) makes the tooth-bone-ulcer bigger still; this "devitalization" by definition diminishes further the tooth's ability to resist infection, although by this time trying to "save" a tooth with a dead core, a fundamentally dead tooth, is nonsense.

   As the entire tooth is being transformed into a pathogenic nest, the infection is spreading through the joint that connects it with the jawbone, and beyond, into the jaw and circulation. The early and persistent infection of the joint between tooth and jaw, and continual leakage into the bloodstream, provides a ready explanation for chronic joint disease, which has been linked to oral focal infections for more than two millennia in any case.

   And all the while, the jawbone is being eaten away by a related chronic, progressive, bone infection. The persistence of secondary jawbone infections, even after all instigating, diseased teeth have been removed, may be a major factor in the persistence of various systemic disease conditions caused by infections emanating from the teeth in the first instance.

   In conclusion, this is not quackery. This is dentistry.

Part III: *PhD Annex -- Defense, and Offense**

Petitioner: Stuart Hale Shakman
Institution: American Academy of Biological Dentistry (AABD)

Degree Title: Doctor of Philosophy in History of Dentistry

Dissertation Title: Medicine's Grandest Fraud -- Revelations of
A Critical Review of Dentistry in the Twentieth Century

    This dissertation wholly incorporates *Parts I & II* above,
previously distributed under the preliminary title *Fraud and Root
Canals*, plus the supporting materials below.

    This dissertation also prominently cites a comprehensive
associated compilation entitled *REFERENCE MANUAL ROSENOW ETAL*.

                    * * * * * * *

CONTENTS:

*This annex of supplementary documentation was submitted 21 June
1999; PhD signed 7 July 1999.

Section 1. Introductory

a. Scope

The central thesis of this dissertation is that a misrepresentation of E.C. Rosenow's otherwise-irreproachable JAMA-published data, by rival bacteriologist W. Holman in 1928, was a defining moment in the history of dentistry -- and indeed the whole of medicine -- with continuing broad implications. This compilation of supplementary substantive documentation was submitted 21 June 1999 as requested by Dr. Arana on behalf of the AABD. (Non-substantive documentation, submitted in accord with PhD guidelines as per Encyclopedia Britannica and Turabian, is incorporated as Part 9. General PhD Criteria.)

The substantive materials presented are attributable to the petitioner and do not represent endorsement by the AABD, or vice-versa, although there is general and fundamental agreement on the harmful systemic effects of persistent oral ("focal") infections.

While it is hoped that this submission may set a properly rigorous precedent for potential future other action by the AABD, it is recognized that its utility at best would be from a general rather than specific perspective. Given the necessarily individual and advanced nature of work at the PhD level, specific questions pertaining to a given dissertation would tend not to have wider applicability. This is particularly true of historical scholarship as compared to scientific.

As Sarton has noted, whereas scientific preparation must be carried on in a certain order, e.g. algebra before analysis, chemistry before physiology, etc., "it is possible ... to study history in almost any order, and the majority of scholars have obtained their historical knowledge in the most haphazard way. One may be an expert in American history and know nothing whatever of the Sumerians or the Hittites." (The Study of the History of Science, G. Sarton, Dover 1957, p. 7.)

In the case of dentistry, even the term history may be variously defined. For example, reference to dental disease may be traced a Sumerian civilization which existed as early as 5000 BC, and reference to oral focal infection is seen as early as Assyrian medical records of the 7th Century B.C.; however, the birth of dentistry as a distinct entity occurred much more recently, and is generally attributed to "Father of Dentistry" Pierre Fauchard in the 18th Century, and it was not until a century later, in America, that the first school dedicated to the study of dentistry was founded.

This dissertation is primarily and intensively concerned with the subsequent critical and pivotal modern/American period in the history of dentistry, with emphasis on the first half of the 20th Century; however, implications on understanding the history of dentistry (and health science overall) from the broadest of perspectives, dating back to the very beginning of civilization as we know it, are also and necessarily incorporated.

Section 1. b. Overview Q. & A.

Question (1):
   Can historical works re-emerge as truly significant?

Answer (1):
   Nature 338, 456, "Heliocentric tangents", authored by the petitioner, illustrated how discoveries may languish for long periods prior to becoming generally known, e.g., 1800 years in the case of the heliocentric hypothesis. It is therefore not unprecedented, though nonetheless disappointing, that the definitive bacteriological works of Rosenow, et al. have for the present slipped into relative obscurity.

Question (2):
   What is the place of the history of modern dentistry within the contexts of the history of the focal infection concept and the history of medicine?

Answer (2):
   Pivotal. The main thrust of modern dentistry, particularly during the last half of the 20th Century and with the full collusion and even encouragement of modern medicine, has tended to isolate dental considerations from medical ones, served to suppress consideration of the focal infection concept, and thereby served to subvert medical progress. Underlying issues strike at the very heart of the state of medicine at the start of the 21st Century, and resolution is indispensably critical to the future of medicine, These subjects are addressed in greater detail in Parts I and II above, particularly in Part I - Preface and Chapter (1); and Part II, Appendix K.

Question (3):
   What is the nature of the major historical event treated in this petition?

Answer (3):
   In contrast to seemingly more common instances of fabrication of data associated with scientific fraud, this study involves an instance of an intricate scheme to discredit valid research results. (See Part I. <2>, above).

Question (4):
   How is this dissertation to be distinguished from garden-variety "fraud and conspiracy" theories?

Answer (4):
   There is nothing theoretical about the central thesis of this dissertation. The deceptive scheme exposed herein was too intricate to be accidental, and did in fact misrepresent Rosenow's results. Details of Holman's clear-cut bastardization of Rosenow's irreproachable research results are set forth in

Part I <3>, above.

Question (5):
   What are broader implications, particularly related to the development of dentistry in the mid 20th Century?

Answer (5):
   The entirety of "scientific" justification in support of the practice of root canal "therapy" (a truly super-oxymoronic concept) is fatally flawed, exposing the frailty of foundations of the whole of modern dental practice. Such implications are discussed in Part I <4> and <5>.

Question (6):
   Certainly one alleged fraudulent article does not in-and-of-itself warrant disregarding modern endodontics. ... Well, does it?

Answer (6):
   No, but it does bring into question a body of subsidiary literature that weighed heavily and essentially in support of proliferation of the practice of endodontics (root canal procedures). In contrast, every properly conducted study has reaffirmed that the practice of devitalizing teeth makes an already-bad situation even worse. (See Part I <6>, above) All non-vital teeth are infected. It is possible that the future will find that the single major contributing factor in the current cancer epidemic is endodontics.
   For example, according to the 1990 ADA Survey of Dental Services Rendered, Table 15, root canal procedures more than doubled (percentage-wise) and extractions more than halved in 1979 compared to 1959. And according to U.S. PHS #96-1232, incidences of some cancers as of 1992 were 2.5 times the 1973 levels (e.g. prostate cancer in white males and lung cancer in white females). (See "The Oncodontistry Epidemic, 2000 AD", Section 3, below).

Question (7):
   Cancer? You must be joking. Realistically, how extensive are implications on medicine as a result of Holman's action?

Answer (7):
   As demonstrated by Rosenow, et al., virtually all mysterious chronic, and even acute, diseases may entail complicity of an infected oral focus, except for the likes of entities involving an identifiable vector (e.g. malaria). A list of disease entities discussed by Rosenow is provided in Part I, Appendix A.
   Extending these to cancer, for example, we know that stomach ulcers are secondary to oral foci, and that stomach cancer (when it occurs) follows stomach ulcers. Therefore, insofar as the initial inciting cause has been demonstrated to be oral foci, there is logic in the suggestion that toxins associated with the

end stage of life in the oral focus might be a primary
contributor to the end stage of life (i.e. cancer) in the
secondary disease location.

   Beyond reproducing a wide range of specific disease symptoms
in laboratory animals with IV injections, the work of Rosenow and
associates involved a number of other tests which were presented
as further support of proof of etiology, including: induction
with streptococci of foci in teeth in dogs; cataphoretic studies;
diagnostic cutaneous tests; precipitation reaction with blood
serum and antiserum; and agglutination tests.

   Numerous investigators have replicated Rosenow's work in a
wide range of disease conditions [e.g., 15 citations are listed
on p. A2-23; several thousand experiments by Rosenow and 31
others are summarized in Table 2.1 on p. 2.1 of *REFERENCE MANUAL
ROSENOW ET AL*; and a number of enthusiastic testimonials are
found in the literature, e.g. Rowntree's account of how Rosenow
was able to repeatedly "set off syndromes in rabbits [which were]
the exact counterparts of the clinical manifestations observed in
the patients - especially tics of one kind or another" [section
1.2, pp. 1-4 to 1-5 of *REFERENCE MANUAL ROSENOW ET AL.*]

Question (8):
   If Rosenow's work was so substantial, why is there so little
in the public record regarding its value?

Answer (8):
   On the contrary, numerous testimonials are to be found in the
historical record. See Part I. Appendix B, above. And beyond
these glowing reports is a mountainous body of irrefutable and
consistent work by numerous investigators demonstrating that the
method of Rosenow has indeed fulfilled the venerable Koch-Henle
criteria for proof of disease causation. Rosenow himself
published some 300 articles in the medical literature, including
38 in JAMA. (In a very real sense, the rest of medicine is much
like the proverbial chicken that keeps running around after its
head has been cut off. Or like the proverbial first "king" in
"The king is dead; long live the king.")

Question (9):
   Are there reasons, beyond Holman's action, for the continued
obscurity of the works of Rosenow et al.?

Answer (9):
   Common arguments against Rosenow, and proposed rebuttals
gleaned from his works, are discussed in Part I, Appendices <C>
and <D> above. Among these, a 1938 article by Cecil and Angevine
is of particular continuing interest in that it is prominently
cited in the public literature in opposition to the concept of
focal infection. See also Question (14) and Section 4, below,
for further discussion of the Cecil and Angevine article.

   These articles have certainly played a major contributing role
reinforcing a general perception, without specific reasons given,

that Rosenow's work is invalid.

Question (10):
   How did this perception spread through the historical
literature, and what was the position of Louis Grossman, who is
generally acknowledged as the father of modern endodontics?

Answer (10):
   Although not one of the founding members of the American
Association of Endodontics, Grossman's activism and longevity
played a major role in the ascendance of endodontics as a
discipline of dentistry domestically and abroad. His published
textbooks on the subject spanned the incredible period of 1940
through 1988, and translations into a number of languages enabled
the spread of this practice worldwide.
   The progression of anti-Rosenow sentiment through the
endodontics and dental literature, in particular, and Grossman's
apparently key role in this, is discussed in Part I, Appendix E.
and Part II, Appendix F, above. It is noted, however, that
throughout his career even Grossman had insisted on assuring the
sterility of the root canal before filling, a requirement that
authorities in modern endodontics (e.g. Seltzer) has (a)
acknowledged as not possible and (b) consequently ignored.

Question (11):
   What were the pre-conditions that contributed to this
situation, and how does this relate to the essential early
history of modern dentistry?

Answer (11):
   These pre-conditions date all the way back to the earliest
times in recorded history. Within the longer-range multi-
millennia historical perspective, one might easily and properly
characterize 20th century enshrinement of endodontics as the
clear culmination and continuation the ancient legend of the
tooth worm. The process of extirpating the pulp from the
interior of the tooth is incomprehensible from a modern 21st (or
even 19th or 20th) century physiological perspective, and wholly
sensible only, and readily, from that of the fabled tooth worm.
(See Section 6, below, "Legend of the Toothworm, 5000 BC - 2000
AD.")
   Factors contributing to perpetuation of the tooth worm
hypothesis in modern times, including the particularly central
role of former ADA President and longtime JADA editor C. N.
Johnson (also former Dean of the Chicago College of
Dentistry/Loyola, the dental school attended by Dr. George Meinig
DDS) are discussed in Part II, Appendix G, above.
   In large part, general opposition of dentistry to Rosenow et
al. can be largely attributed to an inherent conflict of interest
-- the understandable inability of sworn (albeit however sincere
and well-intentioned) tooth-savers to be totally objective on the
question of whether compromised teeth can be saved at all. The

logical extension of the Rosenow et al. position entails the
necessary rejection of the bulk of not merely modern dental
practice but the total demise of the continuing influence of the
legend of the tooth worm. This has clearly not yet occurred.

Question (12):
   Given dentistry's acknowledged good intentions of saving
teeth, how can the petitioner dare to suggest that the legacy of
modern dentistry may redefine quackery?

Answer (12):
   That is a good question. If, for example, a quack need not be
aware that his own practice is indeed quackery, then modern
dentistry could simply be regarded as merely the worst and latest
of the genre. However, for reasons discussed in Part II,
Appendix K, above, the insidious harmfulness of modern dentistry
seems to warrant enshrinement as a transcendent category of
improper action.
   It is further noted that the modern position is far more
extreme, in terms of "saving teeth", than that of Pierre
Fauchard, the "Father of Dentistry". Some highlights of
Fauchard's work are provided in Section 7,below, "Pierre
Fauchard, Father of Dentistry".

Question (13):
   As raised by Dr. David Kennedy, DDS, at the 1999 AABD meeting,
at what point is a carious tooth beyond saving?

Answer (13):
   As viewed from the perspective of any other open wound to the
protective surface of the human body, full healing and salvation
(of the tooth) are intimately intertwined. As Martin Fischer,
M.D., emphasized some six decades ago, aptly describing the
situation even today as we move into a new millennium, we still
don't know how to reverse caries and regenerate compromised tooth
bone (dentin and enamel).
   In *Death and Dentistry* (1940), Fischer had provided a
masterful review, validation and extension of the works of Frank
Billings, E.C. Rosenow and others, from the physiological
perspective. All types of systemic diseases were discussed as
secondary to oral focal infections, with particular emphasis on
residual jawbone infections as a causative focus, and the need
for surgical intervention. He also emphasized how organisms
infecting different types of tissue within the oral focus will
tend to infect similar types of tissue elsewhere in the body,
primarily sown through the bloodstream. (See also Section 5,
below.)
   On the subject of extractions, I am fully in accord with
Fischer's opposition to extraction of any and all "perfectly good
teeth". But those that are compromised beyond any reasonable hope
of ever fully healing, given their proven systemic implications,
would appear to be logical candidates for extraction. It is

hoped that at least some middle-aged teeth, despite Fischer's pessimistic assessment of such teeth in general, may both externally and x-ray-roentenographically fit Fischer's definition of "perfectly good teeth", in which case they would preferably be retained.

Question (14):
   But even one of Rosenow's close early associates, Cecil, had a change of mind about the value of this work. Isn't that proof that it deserves to be forgotten?

Answer (14):
   It is true that Cecil and Angevine's 1938 article is often cited, e.g. on a current British Dental Association web page, as evidence that Rosenow's work is passé. However, an actual reading of this 1938 article shows this not to be the case. An assessment of this issue is provided in Section 4, below.

Question (15):
   Don't dentists know more about the teeth than anyone else?

Answer (15):
   Yes they do, in the same sense that a caterpillar is intimately knowledgeable of the leaf on which it feeds. But as for knowledge of the forest, or even the tree or its branch, we must consult with the likes of Martin Fischer and facts of physiology. See Section 5, below.

Question (16):
   How about the anatomical perspective? Didn't Gray ("Gray's Anatomy") show how teeth are an outgrowth of the skin, and hence more like a fingernail than a bone?

Answer (16):
   Yes and no. Although Gray discussed how the teeth appear to be generated from the dermoid system, the womb of the teeth is obviously a very specialized type of "skin" -- otherwise we'd have teeth sprouting from all areas of the skin. Rather, as Fischer and others have shown, the tooth once developed is for all practical purposes a bone, the enamel is analogous to a hoof (or fingernail or horn as discussed by Fauchard), dentin analogous to bone tissue, and "root" analogous to bone-marrow. Thus, as Fischer offered, a compromised tooth is a compound fracture, physiologically, and only the finding of a method of completely healing it will rectify the situation. This and/or the cloning of bona fide replacement teeth, must top the list of goals of biological dentistry in the coming millennium.

Question (17):
   Now that you have trashed modern dentistry, what conclusions are to be drawn for the teaching of the History of Dentistry?

Answer (17):
    The teaching of the History of Dentistry is as relevant and important as it has ever been. As stated by J. Ben Robinson (quoted by Hermann Prinz, Dental Chronology, Lea & Febiger, Phila. 1945): "The dental profession will continue to flounder, to perpetuate its handicaps and to fail to achieve its true purposes as long as it lacks an intelligent understanding of its historical background."
    We may on the one hand take issue with the father of modern dentistry, G.V. Black, for having diverted attention away from the mercury toxicity issue of amalgams (by virtue of having solved the amalgam expansion problem through the use of alloys; see discussion in Section 7 on Fauchard, relating to mercury and G.V. Black, page 3). Yet we are reminded that Black in his last published work within his lifetime referred to and enthusiastically endorsed the recent works of Hunter, Billings, Rosenow and others on the subject of oral focal infection. Unfortunately he was not able to follow up on the full implications of this work, or we would have all have benefited from a kinder and gentler subsequent history of dentistry in the 20th century. G. V. Black's final words on focal infection are incorporated as Section 8, "The Dentist's Opportunity".

Question (18):
    In that this thesis is primarily concerned with health implications of infected oral foci including teeth, rather than dentition, does this properly fall within the proper scope of the History of Dentistry?

Answer (18):
    A range of health-related hypotheses and perspectives, beyond mechanical considerations of dentition, properly fall within the AABD scope, including most prominently its own conceptual approach, which lies at the interface of health and dentistry, i.e., biological dentistry. Indeed, the impetus toward and goal of true and full biocompatibility of any allowable dental intervention is truly the vanguard of the future of health science, and, for better or worse, the AABD apparently its greatest champion at the present time.

Question (19):
    Why is the subject area appropriate for philosophical study on the doctoral level, warranting the award of a doctor of philosophy degree (PhD)?

Answer (19):
    The key conclusion to be drawn from the work is broadly philosophical in nature, with implications for the overall history of health science -- demanding no less than elevation of consideration of health implications of oral focal infections to primary position within the scope of dentistry, decisively above cosmetic considerations, and the harnessing of the indispensable

and unique technical capabilities of dentistry (as well as any and all appropriate disciplines and capabilities of medicine) in support of such a scope. At a minimum this would seemingly involve full reintegration of dentistry within medicine as an integral and continuing role at the earliest point of intake, and encompassing essential considerations of prevention, diagnosis, therapy and surgery.

Question (20):
   What promise might the likes of modern progress in stem cell transplantation hold for the resolution of the problem of the wounded tooth bone?

Answer (20):
   A couple observations:
   a. In that stem cells are in the circulating blood (and are in fact commonly being harvested and used in place of marrow-derived cells in transplantation), conceptually one might consider some sort of autoblood-calcium/phosphorus, etc. matrix as the fully "biologically compatible" filling of the future -- one that leads to full healing of the wounded tooth. Such a desirable result would also require resolution of such problems as protection from internal as well as external assault during the healing process.
   b. In the meantime, given our present state of knowledge, the surest and safest course of action would appear to be to follow Fischer's recommendation of getting rid of all hopelessly compromised teeth (i.e. all teeth that will not fully heal) before they get rid of us. It is admittedly very difficult to embrace such a position, which is readily labeled "extreme" in the current "intellectual" climate thanks to the incredible amount of brainwashing we have all received to the contrary. But both logic and science firmly validate the Fischer view. Neither our best intentions nor the passage of time will alter these facts; rather we can serve either to accelerate awareness of them, or as formerly unwitting agents of continued repression.

Question (21):
   How might the works of Rosenow et al. be related to modern methods of testing for infections in teeth, e.g., the methodology of Dr. Boyd Haley at the U. of Ky. for measuring toxicity of "avital" teeth and jawbone infections?

Answer (21):
   At a minimum, use of the Rosenow methodology can serve as a test for validation of the Haley results. Following protocols established by Rosenow, a number of investigators have concluded that most or even all non-vital teeth are infected -- this with the organism demonstrated to be etiologically related to a wide range of systemic diseases by Dr. Rosenow and others. (For example, see Part I. <6>, above; and discussions of Haden 1928, pages B2-14-15 of REFERENCE MANUAL ROSENOW ET AL.) Accordingly,

the testing of teeth by Rosenow's methods may help assure that suspect teeth absolved by other methods do not nonetheless harbor harmful bacteria and thus be candidates for extraction.

For specific example, some comparison of Rosenow cultures from AD patients v. controls may provide useful data to augment Haley's results with AD, insofar as Dr. Rosenow's so-cultured organisms were noted to remarkably replicate neurological symptoms in some conditions (e.g. see para. <1.2> in *REFERENCE MANUAL ROSENOW ET AL*).

And the Rosenow methodology also yields a therapeutic vaccine that has been highly praised.

It seems worthy of noting the "coincidence" that Dr. Haley's work involves the use of the third "wash" or "extraction" for testing of toxicity, in that, from about 1935 through the late 1950s, E.C. Rosenow developed and used a serial dilution method to isolate strains of organisms for culturing and use in animal experimentation, other tests, and in vaccines. Rosenow's final method involved use of a third dilution, explaining that lesser dilutions allowed other organisms to crowd out the finicky ones that were really causing the damage. Rosenow's serial dilution method is described further in the above-cited compilation on Rosenow, Chapter <4>,

Question (22):
How might Dr. Jerry Bouquot's contemporary characterization of "bone marrow edema", as may be applied to jawbone infections, relate to Fischer's extensive writings on the subject of edemas?

Answer (22):
In a 1939 article on Edema in G. M. Piersol's Cyclopedia of Medicine, Fischer characterized a wide range of ills as edemas, e.g., heart disease, nephritis, diabetes, glaucoma. (Fischer had previously written a textbook on the subject of *Edema and Nephritis*; 3rd Ed. 1921.) At the very end of the piece, Fischer traced all of these diverse conditions to a common origin in oral foci. But nowhere (that I have seen) did Fischer refer to infection within the inciting oral focus as edema.

Bouquot's characterization of bone marrow edema within the inciting oral focus, specifically infected jawbone tissue, extends the picture brilliantly. This leads to the question regarding possible (or even logical) extension of such a concept to the tooth itself, with potentially valuable implications for the study of long-term effects of tooth fillings (Fischer opposed any and all). In other words, in that tooth is bone, albeit the hardest in the body as per Fauchard, might the concept of bone marrow edema be extended to infection within the tooth bone itself?

Question (23):
How might current work relating trigeminal neuralgia to oral foci be correlated with the works of the earlier writers?

Answer (23):

It is noted that not long after the period referred to in a contemporary review as the "first Golden Age of Dentistry" (1835-1860) [Bouquot and Lense, *Oral Surgery...*, Sept. 1994], Dr. Austin Flint's 1868 prominent medical textbook related trigeminal neuralgia ("formerly called tic douloureaux") to caries: " ... An occasional cause of this condition is caries of the teeth. It is by no means frequently referable to this cause, but that it is so occasionally cannot be doubted." (Flint would serve as 36th President of the AMA in 1886.)

Fischer's view a half-century later was more definite, asserting that trifacial neuralgias and facial tics most commonly are secondary to primary infection in the teeth [*Death and Dentistry*, 1940, p. 169], noting also that the nerve in the tooth-pulp is a branch of the trigeminus [p. 59].

E. C. Rosenow, MD, head of experimental bacteriology at Mayo from 1915-1944, reported that organisms from dental and other foci, taken from persons with trigeminal neuralgia, electively produced lesions of the gasserian ganglion and branches of the facial nerves in laboratory animals; and recommended: "The removal of foci in instances of trigeminal neuralgia (and in my experience their presence is constant in this condition) obviously should be done as a preventive measure before central irreversible lesions have occurred ... ". [See E.C. Rosenow, 1940 ADA Centennial, p. 271, reprinted in the *REFERENCE MANUAL ROSENOW ET AL*, A5-B; and A4, 53R1.] Rosenow's observations seem to be substantially in accord with Bouquot's reference to three studies in the 1970s indicating "laboratory evidence of gasserian ganglion demyelination after damage as far away as a tooth pulp" [Bouquot, et. al., *Oral Surgery...*, March 1992].

Question (25):

In that the Rosenow and Fischer works implicated microbial infection as the cause of systemic infection secondary to oral foci, including neurological disease, what might be the relation to theories relating to neural transmission of disease, and associated implications for therapy?

Answer (25):

Fischer may be interpreted as contraindicating the views of a modern European "movement", reflected in the works of Issels and others in the U.S., to the extent they are associated with the theory of neural transmission of systemic disease and the sometimes-associated practice of injecting anesthesia, particularly into nerves. The contrary Fischer view from the perspective of the health of nerve tissue that may be so injected finds support in some contemporary views questioning the safety of such procedures, e.g., as communicated to the petitioner by Steve Evans DDS and of Lowell Weiner DDS, Capital U. of Integrative Med., and others.

It is not readily clear how, or even if, Fischer's (et. al.) and Issels's (et. al.) views on the theory of neural transmission may be reconciled, but in any case the Fischer position, supported by the incredible mass of documentation of E.C. Rosenow, Weston Price and their many associates, is unassailable. Moreover, Rosenow's work establishes an intimate relation between bacterial infection and allergic and toxic phenomena; and fulfills the venerable Koch-Henle criteria for disease causation; all of which might arguably further isolate the neural perspective, on which the burden of reconciliation would appear to fall, on the basis that "more is in vain when less will serve" (Newton, Mathematical Principles). In this regard, there are some practical as well as theoretical considerations derivable from autotherapeutical and Fischer/Rosenow perspectives, including proposed tests, implicated modifications, comparisons, etc. (It must be noted that notwithstanding the above-discussed difference on the "neural" issue, Issels et al. are in broad agreement with the Fischer/Rosenow perspective in condemnation and need for removal of oral infections as a major factor in combating systemic disease.)

Question (26):
    How might this "neural issue" be reconciled with the observation of unrelated successful intervention mechanisms?

Answer (26):
    This does not mean to deny the possibility that interventions via mechanisms that otherwise are not in-and-of-themselves specifically causative may nonetheless yield genuine therapeutic benefits attributable to impact on actual causative factors. There is also the possibility that first-level symptoms may find themselves being characterized as causative in situations where their (derivative) connection with actual first cause is not evident.

Question (27):
    What are implications for the complementary/integrative medical approach?

Answer (27):
    The full realization of the unanimity and impregnability of the proofs of the role of oral infections (incorporating derivative conditions of toxicity and allergy) in the etiology of a cornucopian preponderance of systemic diseases (by Rosenow, Billings, Fischer, Price, Haden, etc.) seemingly demands a soul-searching reassessment of more recent alternative perspectives and approaches (including even modern immunology theory) from that fundamental and encompassing perspective. In that the proofs of Rosenow et al. are complete, irrefutable and comprehensive, it seems inevitable that this work will become the "medical guide of the future" as predicted by AMA President Walter Bierring 60 years ago. This does not mean that the work cannot be improved and extended, and this may indeed come through some other work currently being conducted within the scope of

contemporary integrative medicine. But the situation seems to
call for using the Rosenow-Fischer et al. position as the
starting point for an integrative effort, rather than viewing it
as one of many competing or even complementary approaches.

     And at a minimum, Rosenow's work comprises a framework for
testing the impact of other types of interventions on the
bacteriological and associated (e.g. toxic), arguably causative
factors, e.g. tests involving electrophoresis, specific antigen
and/or antibody reactions.

Question (28):
     What are specific implications for dentistry?

Answer (28):
     Pervasive, if indeed tooth is bone as asserted by
authorities since the 18th Century, e.g., "father of dentistry"
Pierre Fauchard and "master of comparative anatomy" John Hunter
(as per Donald T. Atkinson, 1956, p. 188); and if indeed all
filled or otherwise compromised teeth are properly viewed as
compound fractures, as Fischer in particular so strongly
asserted.
     From such a perspective, issues such as relative
biocompatibility, toxicity and oral galvanism, however important
they may be with reference to filled teeth, seem clearly
secondary. In this regard, the need for assessing the pathology
of tooth tissue under fillings relative to that of jawbone and
other bone tissue, as discussed above, assumes both relative and
absolute significance.
     Likewise, if the very fact of even-minimally compromised
teeth is definitive as concerns continued existence of (focal)
infection, seemingly indicating a need for earliest possible
removal (if no longer fully healable or containable) and/or
specific Rosenowian vaccine-therapy, what is the proper place for
other categories of diagnosis and therapy? This is not to say
that these others do not have a place, but rather that their role
might well be clarified relative (secondary) to the work Rosenow
et al., the central role of oral focal infections, and associated
implications.

Question (29):
     What are associated implications for medicine?

Answer (29)
     In his often-quoted 1913 presentation to the Chicago Dental
Society, entitled "Constitutional Diseases Secondary To Local
Infections", Charles H. Mayo asserted that virtually all diseases
are caused by infectious agents, and that most of these must come
from oral foci. This is why he concluded, "The next great step
in medical progress in the line of preventive medicine should be
made by the dentists." He was not calling on the dentists for
more research or independent new initiatives, although certainly
much that has since occurred along these lines would have been

welcomed. Rather, he was clearly calling for direct action when
he issued his challenge -- to a top-ranking *dental* audience --
"The question is will they do it?"

    Except for the names of the participants, the ensuing
discussion could have been conducted in Carmel in 1999 -- or
2001: Arthur D. Black referred to the "important role which
mouth infections play as causative factors of lesions elsewhere
in the body." James B. Herrick discussed how toxins emanating
from foci gradually infect joint, nerve, or other tissue over a
period of years. D. J. Davis appealed to dentists to furnish
material from mouth infections to pathologists and
bacteriologists. W. E. Post referred to neurasthenia, neuritis
and lumbago as having a toxic origin with toxins coming from oral
bacterial infections. M.L. Rhein called for anaerobic
bacteriological examination of material from chronic alveolar
abscess. Frederick B. Moorehead offered "Bone cavities in the
jaws may be present for years unknown in the patient." Edward C.
Rosenow spoke of the mechanism of endocarditis as "an embolic
process." And Thomas B. Hartzell, who would later serve as ADA
President, referred to Mayo's "epoch-marking paper for dentistry"
with the admonition that "We must take heed or we will be
stranded among the artisans instead of taking our proper place in
the medical world."

    Further, since Rosenow et al. long ago showed that oral
focal infections cause diseases later termed "autoimmune",
ignoring Rosenow's earlier work, where does this leave the modern
science of immunology and "immune system" theory which evolved in
concert with the "autoimmunity" concept (e.g. I. Roitt,
Immunology, 1970), and how severely does this weaken arguments
based on it?

Question (30)
    At what stage in the process of tooth decay does infection
reach the root, and what are implications?

Answer (30):
    This apparently occurs relatively early in the infection
process, an alarming prospect insofar as such a progression is
generally considered irreversible. Six years following Mayo's
historic plea to dentists, Hartzell, with Henrici, followed with
a "epoch-marking" paper of their own, less well-known than Mayo's
but perhaps no less significant, "The Bacteriology of Vital
Pulps" (J. Dent. Res. 1919, p. 419-422). They observed that
streptococcal infection had already reached the pulp in about
half of (103) vital teeth with caries and/or pyorrhea, versus
absolutely zero in (22) entirely normal teeth, a result they
termed "startling. ... It is to be remembered that all were
clinically vital teeth with grossly normal pulps." They
concluded that "invasion and destruction of the pulp is
frequently a long drawn out process, microorganisms being present
long before actual necrosis of the tissues takes place."
    Thus is found yet additional authoritative inspiration and

support for inclusion within the scope of modern dental inquiry, beyond the question of how best to save compromised teeth, of the question of whether (or past what point) such teeth can be saved at all. In this regard the AABD seems to be alone among peers in inclusion of such a fundamental question within its scope via the likes of Fischer's "Death and Dentistry".

It is acknowledged that this issue strikes at the very heart of what much of dentistry has become (e.g. Hartzell had cautioned against dentists becoming mere "artisans"), but on reflection it does not necessarily render the "biological dentistry" portion of the AABD title "an oxymoron". Rather it seems to call for refining the focus and definition of dentistry in terms of what it must increasingly become in the future -- the true leading edge of medicine, both preventive in the long term as envisaged by Mayo, and aggressively curative in the short term as eloquently illustrated and discussed by Fischer. This would seem to mandate that the medical examination of the future begin with a thorough dental examination, and that dentistry's goal of "saving teeth" at all costs take a back seat to a new mission of "saving health and life". And the public must be educated as to the clear choice between saving one's health and saving one's teeth in cases where teeth are irreversibly compromised.

The bottom line is that medical doctors simply don't have the tools to address this root cause of systemic disease, so the dentists will have to do it.

Section 2: Technical Abstract

Technical notes: This abstract is in letter form as it was first submitted as correspondence to Nature in October 1993. It was returned by Executive Editor Maxine Clarke (SHAKMAN COMM/MC/tb, 2 November 1993) with the suggestion it be sent to a clinical journal as it seemed to not be of "compelling interest" to Nature. It was accordingly submitted but not published in JAMA (#JLD71261, 12 Dec. 97). Subsequently, it was independently reviewed by Dr. Clarence Williamson, former Dean of Biological Studies at Miami U., Oxford, Ohio, and associate of the late Dr. Martin Fischer, M.D. Dr. Williamson was also apparently the last investigator to regularly produce E.C. Rosenow's vaccines; he enthusiastically endorsed the information in the abstract and expressed disappointment that JAMA had not published it.

Abstract of Dissertation:

Subject: Doctoring the numbers - medicine's greatest fraud
To the Editor. --
    This letter exposes a fraudulent scheme, introduced in a letter to this journal by W. L. Holman with details published elsewhere[1]; which was apparently specifically intended to discredit prominent research results published in this journal by Edward C. Rosenow and in former A.M.A. President Frank Billings' associated work[2], and broad and continuing implications.
    Rosenow, head of experimental bacteriology for the Mayo Foundation from 1915-1944, published nearly 300 articles (including 45 in this journal) over the period 1902-1958. His animal experiments repeatedly demonstrated the phenomenon of "elective localization", whereby organisms isolated from dental and other foci of persons with a wide range of diseases were found to have a specific affinity for corresponding tissues when injected into laboratory animals. Billings suggested that cells in these tissues adsorb the bacteria out of the circulation "as if by a magnet".[2]
    For example, Rosenow found that 60% of 103 animals injected with bacteria from stomach ulcer patients developed stomach or duodenal hemorrhages, compared with 17% of 405 animals injected with other strains. Holman calculated from Rosenow's data that such lesions had developed in 62 of the former ("specific") vs. 68 of the latter ("non-specific") instances, performed the same sort of calculations with Rosenow's other data (Table 1), and carefully stated that it is "a 50 percent chance" that any particular localization is due to a "specific' or 'non-specific" strain. Based on this faulty and essentially meaningless construction, he referred to Rosenow's elective location hypothesis as "a theory with little if any experimental basis" and dismissed Rosenow's experimental results as "unconvincing".[1]
    The continuing broad significance of Holman's deception is exemplified in Paul Beeson's 1976 authoritative assessment of American medicine[4]. Beeson asserted that the focal infection

work of Rosenow and Billings had been disproved in 1940 by Reimann and Havens.[5] Reimann and Havens, in turn, exclusively credited Holman's 1928 article with having negated Rosenow's animal experiments.

Holman's handiwork also is widely cited in the foundational dental literature underlying the common modern dental practice of retaining devitalized teeth (which Rosenow vehemently opposed), as for example perpetuated through the lasting legacy of Louis I. Grossman[6], which in turn continues to contribute to modern opposition to the focal infection concept in general.

At the 1940 Dental Centenary Celebration, Rosenow presented results of experiments involving more than 11,000 animals by 32 investigators including himself (Table 2), and cited confirming studies of precipitation and cutaneous reactions, electrophoretic mobilities, and agglutination and other tests.[3]   In all, the works of Rosenow and associates seem to have gone far beyond merely fulfilling the venerable Koch-Henle criteria of disease causation for a wide range of diverse diseases.

The fact that Rosenow's work has been wrongfully discredited mandates reassessment, including reconsideration of his emphases on the role of oral focal infections and his unique methodology for the preparation and use of autogenous vaccines.

Former A.M.A. President Walter Bierring has firmly asserted that Rosenow's work had been definitely confirmed, and predicted "perchance it is safe to assume that the 'Rosenow heresy' may yet become the medical guide of the future."[7] Perhaps Dr. Bierring's future has arrived.

S. Hale Shakman
1248 Fifth Street
P.O. Box 382
Santa Monica, CA 90406-0382

References:

1.   Holman, WL. The localization in animals of bacteria isolated from foci of infection. *JAMA*. 1927; 88:424-425 (preliminary letter, without details); *Archives Path. & Lab. Med.* 1928; 5:68-136; table on p. 133.

2.   Rosenow, EC. Elective Localization of Streptococci. *JAMA*. 1915; 65:1687-1691, data on p. 1688; data also in Billings, F., *FOCAL INFECTION, The Lane Medical Lectures* (Delivered on Sept. 20-24, 1915), D. Appleton and Co., N.Y. & London, 1916, p. 36.

3.   Rosenow, EC. Focal infection and elective localization in relation to systemic disease: a review and results of further studies. *Dental Centenary Proceedings*, Maryland State Dental Association and the American Dental Association, March 1940, pp. 261-282.

4.   Beeson, PB. Focal infection and systemic disease; in Bowers J, Purcell E, eds., *Advances in American Medicine: Essays at the Bicentennial*, 1. N.Y.:J. Macy Foundation; 1976, pp. 151-2.

5.   Reimann HA, Havens WP. Focal infection and systemic disease: A critical appraisal. *JAMA*. 1940; 114:1-6.

6.   Grossman LI. *Root Canal Therapy*, 1940-1955 (eds. 1-4); continued as *Endodontic Practice*, 1960-1988 (eds. 5-11). Philadelphia; Lea & Febiger.

7.   Bierring WL. Focal infection: Quarter century survey, Frank Billings Lecture. *JAMA*. 1938;111:1623-1627.

Table 1:   ROSENOW'S RESULTS[2] VS. HOLMAN'S "REARRANGEMENT"[1]

(Data shown for bacteria as initially isolated only)

LESIONS IN ANIMALS' \/	SOURCE: PATIENTS WITH \/	Rosenow's Results		Holman's "Rearrangement"	
		ANIMALS INJECTED \/	% WITH* LESIONS \/	ANIMALS WITH LESIONS	%**
Stomach/duod. w/hemorrhages	Stomach ulcer	103	60%	(= 62)	48%
	Other diseases	405***	17%***	(= 68)	52%
				130	
Stomach/duod. with ulcer	Stomach ulcer	103	60%	(= 62)	67%
	Other diseases	405	7%	(= 30)	33%
				92	
Joints	Rheumatic fever	71	66%	(= 47)	36%
	Other diseases	437	19%	(= 84)	64%
				131	
Endocardium	Endocarditis	44	84%	(= 37)	30%
	Rheumatic fever	71	46%	(= 33)	27%
	Other diseases	393	13%	(= 52)	42%
				122	
Myocardium	Rheumatic fever	71	44%	(= 32)	38%
	Myositis	40	35%	(= 14)	17%
	Other diseases	397	9%	(= 36)	44%
				82	

Table 1 (cont.)

Muscles	Rheumatic fever	71	27%	| (= 19)	24%
	Myositis	40	75%	| (= 30)	38%
	Other diseases	397	7%	| (= 29)	37%
				|	78
Gallbladder	Cholecystitis	41	80%	| (= 33)	43%
	Other diseases	467	9%	| (= 43)	57%
				|	76
Appendix	Appendicitis	68	68%	| (= 46)	71%
	Other diseases	440	4%	| (= 19)	29%
				|	65
Kidneys	Rheumatic fever	71	39%	| (= 28)	52%
	Other diseases	437	6%	| (= 26)	48%
				|	54

* Rosenow: Percent of animals injected that show lesions.
** Holman: Of animals with lesions only, percent from specific
vs. nonspecific sources, without reference to numbers injected.
*** Calculated from Rosenow data for 9 separate "other"
categories, involving strains from: appendicitis (6% of 68
animals), plus cholecystitis (29% of 41), rheumatic fever (23% of
71), erythema nodosom (10% of 20), herpes zoster (29% of 61),
mumps (21% of 19), myositis (4% of 40), myocarditis (7% of 44),
and miscellaneous (17% of 41); or a total of 68 of 405 animals in
all, or 17%. Holman had to perform 36 such sets of calculations
in the course of deriving his "rearrangement".

Table 2. ELECTIVE LOCALIZATION OF STREPTOCOCCI-11,479 ANIMALS [4]

LESIONS IN ANIMALS'	SOURCE: DENTAL/OTHER FOCI IN PERSONS WITH	ROSENOW		ELEVEN CO-WORK.		TWENTY OTHERS		TOTALS	
		#	%	#	%	#	%	#	%
Stomach	Stomach/duodenum ulcer	1539	65	1231	52	280	60	3050	57
	Other diseases	3341	8	1798	6	996	3	6135	06
	No systemic disease	1329	14	665	7	300	7	2294	11
Joints	Arthritis	1447	53	1225	58	415	59	3087	56
	Other diseases	3433	13	1804	7	861	39	6098	15
	No systemic disease	1329	18	665	11	300	31	2294	18
Eyes	Iritis, other eye dis.	272	42	328	43	186	53	786	45
	Other diseases	4608	1	2701	1	1090	1	8399	01
	No systemic disease	1329	8	665	0	300	2	2294	05
Myocardium	Myocarditis	36	61	39	38	94	59	169	54
	Other diseases	4844	3	2990	7	1182	11	9016	06
	No systemic disease	1329	6	665	3	300	17	2294	07
Muscles	Myositis	891	72	50	58	86	56	1027	70
	Other diseases	3989	6	2979	9	1190	12	8158	08
	No systemic disease	1329	3	665	7	300	13	2294	05
Kidneys	Pyelonephritis	168	73	96	83	96	58	360	72
	Other diseases	4712	6	2933	3	1180	16	8825	07
	No systemic disease	1329	9	665	7	300	19	2294	10
Colon	Ulcerative colitis	527	58	60	60	119	42	706	56
	Other diseases	4353	2	2969	0	1157	1	8479	01
	No systemic disease	1329	5	665	0	300	0	2294	03
	TOTALS	6209		3694		1576		11479	

Section 3. The Onco-Endo Epidemic, 2000 AD

As discussed in Questions (7) and (8) in Section 2, above, and beyond the logic of association, striking statistical correlations between cancer and root-canal-procedures are illustrated in below tables:

A. CANCER DATA:

(From Health United States 1995, U.S. Dept. of HHS, DHHS Publ. No. (PHS) 96-1232, p. 169, Table 59, "Age-adjusted cancer incidence rates for selected cancer sites, according to sex and race: Selected geographic areas, selected years 1973-1992", exhibiting numbers of new cases per 100,000 population and annual percent change.)

Table A: Cancer Incidence Rates Estimated annual percentage change, 1973-1992 (all line-items $\geq$1.0% for any one group):

	White Male	Black Male	White Female	Black Female
All sites	1.6	1.8	1.0	1.1
Oral Cavity & pharynx	-.8	1.6		
Esophagus	1.1	.1		
Colon/rectum	.2	1.7		
Colon	.6	1.9		
Rectum	-.5	1.0		
Lung/bronch.	.4	1.1	4.7	4.8
Melanoma of skin			3.4	
Breast			1.8	2.0
Prostate	4.6	3.4		
Urin.bladder	.8	1.1		
Non-Hodgk. Lymphoma	3.8	4.0	2.7	3.9

B. ENDODONTICS DATA

(From 1990 <u>Survey of Dental Services Rendered</u>, June 1994, (c) 1996 ADA)

Table B.1. Percentage of patients receiving selected dental services from private practitioners in the US, by year (from Table 15, p. 25):

	1959	1969	1979	1990
Crowns	1.6	2.9	5.2	5.3
Root Canal Procedures	1.7	2.9	3.2	2.6
Extractions	13.0	9.8	5.4	4.9

Table B.2. Estimates of the total number of selected dental services provided by private practitioners in the US, by year (from Table 16, p. 26):

Crowns, Root canals, Extractions, by private practitioners

	1979	1990
Crowns	15,520,000	34,560,000
Root Canal Procedures	6,790,000	13,870,000
Extractions	52,610,000	46,490,000

"Looking at extractions, root canals, and crowns, it appears that fewer teeth are being extracted and more root canals are being performed, with a crown likely being the final restoration.

Section 4.   Cecil & Angevine 1938 - Review and Analysis
     (CECIL 1938 CLEARLY SUPPORTS FOCAL INFECTION - READ IT!!)

  by S. Hale Shakman, INSTITUTE OF SCIENCE

A review and detailed analysis of Cecil and Angevine, Nov. 1938

  [R.L. Cecil & D.M. Angevine, Ann. Int. Med., 12, November
1938, "Clinical and experimental observations on focal infection,
with an analysis of 200 cases of rheumatoid arthritis"]

  Following Holman's fraudulent article and its derivatives, and
aside from some repeatedly-referenced-by-Grossman not-really
substantial items of Okell & Elliot and Fish & MacLean (intended
to discount the incredible insurmountable irrefutable Billings-
Rosenow legacy on grounds of contamination), the next probably-
key article is one published by Cecil and Angevine in November
1938.

  Cecil and Angevine 1938 is frequently and prominently cited as
having been instrumental in refutation of the concept of focal
infection. The particular significance of this article derives
from Cecil's earlier and strong support of the existence of a
causative relationship between oral focal infection and arthritis
(Cecil and Archer, 1927), and Cecil's now-apparent conversion to
the position of opponent.
  A thorough review of Cecil and Angevine 1938 discloses that it
is a very weak leg indeed, to the extent that modern dentistry is
in part propped up on it, actually lending more in the way of
true support for, rather than refutation of, the Billings-Rosenow
focal infection legacy.

  Cecil and Angevine November 1938 (CA38) seeks to limit
discussion of rheumatoid arthritis, defined as "only those
patients who presented the picture of chronic progressive
inflammatory disease of several joints characterized in the early
stages by periarticular swelling and fusiform fingers, and in the
later stages by ankylosis and deformity."

  A.   CLINICAL PART

  Much (most) of this article, and all of the clinical and major
portion, is retrospective, and clearly and admittedly
speculative:
     1. The article retrospectively referred to Billings's
original 1912 report on 10 arthritis cases, which cases had been
cured or greatly benefited, as "questionable" as to how many were
"typically" rheumatoid. No support or specifics are given.
     2. Then, also retrospectively, CA38 downplays Cecil and
Archer's earlier, 1927, positive results in 200 cases of
arthritis as largely likewise not having been "typical", noting
only 29% had shown fusiform fingers. They concede nonetheless

that cures or improvement had occurred in half of the cases where tonsils were removed and nearly 2/3 of those whose teeth were extracted. No mention was made as to how many of those benefited were "typical" rheumatoid arthritis, so it must be assumed that some portion of those benefited were in fact "typically" rheumatoid. That this is so is further supported by the authors' concession that these earlier results had at the time seemed significant, but asserting that nonetheless "it is possible that a good many cases would have shown improvement even if the foci had not been removed."

3. Finally, we get to the real supposed "meat" of this article, at least according to its title and dominating substance, which also happens to be wholly retrospective and admittedly speculative. This involved "200 cases of rheumatoid arthritis from the records of the private practice of Cecil ... within the last 6 or 7 years. ... No case has been included which did not fulfill the classic pattern of the disease. For example, every case in the series showed, or had shown at some time previously, sever characteristic fusiform fingers ... "

a. In other words, in the first instance, this retrospective construct involved only those in unmistakably advanced stages of disease.

Of these 200 total cases was noted "the sedimentation rate was accelerated in 93% ... and agglutinative reaction with a strain of hemolytic streptococcus was strongly positive in 65%. (This result was noted by Bierring in JAMA 1938 without further discussion except the implication that these are supportive of the concept of streptococcal focal infection and hematogenous dissemination.)

No further identification of the streptococcus was given, e.g. source and strain, history, etc.

b. No subsequent examination of these 200 patients was undertaken, attempted, or anticipated in any form by Cecil and Angevine. Rather it was noted that the records of fully 70% of these cases, at the time of examination by Cecil, had made absolutely no reference at all to the possible existence of any type of focal infection, CA38 simply now asserted that this indicated that no focus had existed at the time of examination. (In retrospect it may be logically offered, that for the Cecil and Angevine retrospective "study" to have admitted otherwise would also have been accusatory of Cecil of having been negligent in his practice.) The authors stated that only 20% of the 200 had had "definite" focal infections and 10% "questionable" ones. The "definite" foci totaled 40 (27 in tonsils, 11 in sinuses, and 2 in teeth); the "questionable", 24 (2 in tonsils, 11 in sinus, 11 in teeth); and 140 were noted as without demonstrable focus; for a total of 204; so there were apparently some duplications among the former two categories. The authors dropped this for now, to return later with slightly different numbers.

c. The authors then sought to divide the 200 cases into two groups, those who gave a prior history of treatment for focal infection, and those that at the time of exam exhibited a focal infection. No indication was given as to whether anyone of the latter group might also have involved prior treatments.

> c.1.   Of the first group it was stated that 92 had previously had tonsils removed, 52 had had at least some teeth extracted, and 12 had been treated for sinusitis. No indication was given as to whether any patients had had more than one type, so the actual number of patients thus referred could have ranged anywhere from 92 to 156, depending on possible duplications. These operations, all completed prior to initial visits with Cecil, had been noted in Cecil's records as having had no effect; except for worsening in the case of 2 operations on tonsils, 3 extractions and 2 sinus operations; temporary improvement in 4 tonsils; and by subtraction benefit in 2 extractions.

Again, this is all based on a retrospective review of Cecil's records concerning treatments occurring before Cecil ever saw the patients.

> c.2.   Regarding the "second group, as of exam by Cecil (over the past 6 or 7 years) focal infections had been observed in 27 tonsils, 11 sinuses and 3 teeth, totaling 41, a slight change from CA38's numbers on a previous page, the 20% (of 200) referred to above in b. Of these, Cecil's records showed that treatments had been given to 20 in the case of tonsils; 5, sinuses; and 3, teeth. No benefits had been recorded except for temporary improvement in the case of 7 tonsils operations.

The authors state that of this group of 200 patients, only 52 had previously had any extractions. There was otherwise absolutely no discussion of the condition of any other teeth of these 48, or of the teeth of the other 148 patients who had had no teeth extracted, except that overall the 200 patients "had exceptionally fine teeth", and "in only 3 cases was additional dentistry performed." In other words, when examined by Cecil over the prior 6-7 years, 98.5% of these 200 patients was noted to require absolutely no dental work, in somewhat sharp contrast to the circumstance that fully 100% of these patients had had fusiform fingers and other indications of "true" rheumatoid arthritis. Again, it seems appropriate to emphasize that not one of these 197 arthritic patients underwent a single dental intervention while in Cecil's care.

The sheer improbability of any random sampling of 200 adults, with or without fusiform fingers, having 98.5% of perfect teeth is so incredible as to enable stating with certainty that this retrospective study involved case reports that clearly did not involve sufficiently careful oral examinations to begin to attempt, on a purely retrospective basis, any meaningful correlations of oral disease with the other disease studied -- rheumatoid arthritis.

Once again, it must be kept in mind that all of CA38 thus far was a retrospective construct based on Cecil's records, which retrospective nonsense comprised far and away the major portion of CA38.

B.   EXPERIMENTAL PART

When we finally reach the actual experimental part of CA38, it is found to be primarily concerned with validating the prior and only tangentially-related research of one of the authors (Angevine) that (1) is not fundamentally concerned with testing the concept of oral focal infection, and (2) in any case nonetheless supportive of its basic tenets, i.e., the role of the oral site as focus, and the significance of the hematogenous route for spreading the infection.

Angevine's prior experiments had supported earlier work of others showing that bacteria injected into skin of previously sensitized animals tended to stay fixed at the site of injection, and did not disseminate from there. In the current series of experiments reported in CA38, this same predominantly negative result was reportedly obtained when "a strain of hemolytic streptococcus" was injected into various types of tissues; at the same time it was recorded that arthritis was in fact produced in more than 10% of the animals, and that the "gums were a particularly favorable site for absorption of bacteria". The percentage correlation of gum injections with production of arthritis was not given but the implication was that it was substantial. (This result is of course totally in accord with the findings of Rosenow and others emphasizing the role of oral foci and difficulty in establishing foci elsewhere).

Using these same bacteria, the authors also produced arthritis in 85% of animals injected intravenously. No specific strain was identified in any of the three locations mentioned in CA38, but interestingly, in Rosenow's subsequent 1940 ADA Centennial article, the organism used by Cecil was specifically discussed as follows (p. 271):

"Cecil and Angevine produced in rabbits, with small doses of streptococci obtained from foci of infection and blood and joint tissues in arthritis, pathologic lesions very similar to those of rheumatoid arthritis in man."

The definiteness of Rosenow's identification leads one to suspect that the specific strain or strains of streptococcus used by Cecil was known to Rosenow and in fact precisely that as so discussed by Rosenow. This seems to some extent confirmed by the gratuitous disclaimer offered by Cecil and Angevine, downplaying the significance of the specific strain of streptococcus used: "it is a well-known fact that arthritis can be readily produced in rabbits by the IV injection of almost any strain of streptococcus". The circumstance that no citations were given to support this "well-known fact" further supports the suggestion that this statement was indeed simply intended to downplay and thus distort the fact that 85% of the animals injected intravenously with the rheumatism strain got rheumatism. Accordingly a strong and probably correct case can be made that the Cecil article really is a forceful validation of the focal infection concept in the case of rheumatoid arthritis.

Finally, in their conclusions the authors downplayed the fact, by omission of reference to it, that the only oral site that was used in their experiments (the gums) was indeed favorable for initiating a focus for both absorption and dissemination of bacteria.

Thus, in summary and conclusion, Cecil and Angevine sought to discredit the entire oral focal infection concept with a combination of (1) confusing and grossly deficient, wholly retrospective, analyses of highly improbable events that had occurred prior to and wholly outside of the care of Cecil; and (2) studies and experiments indicating (a) a non-oral focus was difficult to establish and maintain -- in total agreement with similar findings by Rosenow et. al. and overall a "red herring" (possibly true but irrelevant to the question of oral focal infection), (b) in contrast an oral focus in the gums can be initiated and demonstrated to cause a distant disease, and (c) that rheumatoid arthritis-related streptococci injected into the bloodstream, or implanted in an oral focus and from that entering the circulation, tend to cause rheumatoid arthritis in laboratory animals.

No mention is made anywhere in the article of possible consideration of caries, root therapies, gum disease, or residual jawbone infections in any of the 200 patients, except for the three that were given more dentistry.

Overall, the intent of retrospective study of Cecil's cases might appropriately be viewed as an attempt to further buttress Angevine's work on the difficulty of establishing a non-oral focus, by showing there is no such thing as a focus of infection, It is clear from this analysis that they failed miserably. The shamefulness of their lame construct of clinical-historical-revisionism and bogus experimentation (probably in part a product of academia's "publish-or-perish" mentality; Angevine was at Cornell), is nonetheless overshadowed by that assignable to those advocates of harmful dental practices who continue to cite but obviously have never read CA38. They are urged to do so at the earliest possible convenience, and adjust references to CA38 accordingly. This includes most prominently the British Dental Association (see their web page).

Section 5. Martin Fischer 1940 - Overall Review and Assessment

Martin Fischer - <u>Death and Dentistry</u>, 1940, Charles Thomas and Co., Springfield Ill.
Overall Review and Assessment; Detailed Notes and Excerpts

OVERALL REVIEW AND ASSESSMENT

This is a great and very important book -- a must for every dentist, medical doctor, patient or potential patient.

Fischer eloquently reviews the work of Billings and his school, particularly Rosenow, and pronounces the "Billings-Rosenow Syndrome" as responsible for the great bulk of human disease.

Fischer emphatically substantiates the Billings position that more than 99% of human systemic disease is due to chronic infections in tonsils and/or teeth -- usually symptom-less and often very difficult to detect, but always there. (pp. 107-115.)

Fischer carries the Billings-Rosenow work to its logical/scientific conclusion concerning the flawed nature of dentistry. His declaration as a respected physiologist, that the tooth is a bone, is unequivocal and well founded. His consequent albeit-"extreme" position, that all fillings are bad, is hence actually inescapable. Fischer clearly and simply declares that all "root-canals", all fillings, and virtually all the other invasive things dentists do are bad. Fischer concludes that the whole of dentistry is truly an "abortion".

Considerable emphasis is placed on the importance of residual jawbone infections, and the need to excavate not only areas around extracted teeth, down to good bone, but also to remove residual alveolar ridges down to a smooth surface. (This is covered particularly on pp. 136-137 and in case studies.)

Perhaps the most important and somewhat original contribution of Fischer is his indictment of virtually all teeth, and remaining ridges, in the elderly population of the modern world.

In essence, according to Fischer, after decades of bacterial attack through worn-down teeth or at the gum-line, teeth become insidiously-chronically infected. Fischer describes the tell-tale signs of these generally-symptom-less infections, and declares the situation virtually universal after the age of 50 or 60. (pp. 85-87)

It seems kind of ridiculous that these people, perhaps even younger ones, would be urged by Fischer to have some or all of their teeth pulled, even some without previously dentistried teeth or otherwise-obvious caries. That's the bad news.

But the good news is that under such circumstances these people are going to be well-situated to evade the ravages of the wide range of human diseases that come from these quietly-pathogenic oral nests; they'll be a lot healthier and living very much longer. Indeed, with elimination of all Billings-Rosenow-Syndrome streptococcal disease(s), the 150+ year life span is truly within our grasp. So the long process of growing new teeth, through cloning processes yet to be developed, will not be

nearly so intrusive as upon our current absurdly short life-
spans.

   This does not mean that we must abandon dreams of cleaning,
protecting, healing and regenerating compromised tooth-bone in-
vivo. Rather, it is recognition that this admirable goal remains
a dream at our present stage of knowledge in 1999, calling for
attention to the question as to whether future experimentation
along these lines is best conducted on human or animal subjects.

DETAILED NOTES AND EXCERPTS

   The following section of detailed notes and excerpts do not
pretend to be comprehensive; rather, it is hoped these will
provide an incentive for the reader to personally read the
Fischer book in detail to assure access to its full and
delightful content.
   Particular attention in the following notes is paid to the
question of residual jawbone and tonsillar infections, and to
Fischer's position on anesthesia and nervous system
considerations.
   Notwithstanding the temptation to group all "jawbone" notes
with like items, etc., the notes have been left in sequential
order so that they might serve as a guide to a more thorough
reading of the work. Fischer is a terrific writer, very witty,
very enjoyable.
   The book, *Death and Dentistry*, should be available through most
medical libraries; insofar as it is no longer in print, the
American Academy of Biological Dentistry is making available
working copies for educational purposes.

(Caution: Direct quotes from Fischer are so marked; all other
statements are interpretations of the reviewer and thus may vary
from the Fischer view -- all the more reason to read Fischer
directly.)

THE MASTER, FRANK BILLINGS
Book is dedicated "to the memory of the master, Frank Billings"

DENTISTRY BONE SURGERY [Preface]
   In his preface Fischer defines dentistry as bone surgery,
performed for the most part in the face of infection. Fischer
asserts that this requires a drastic revision of all dentistry,
as had been advocated by him and associates 25 years earlier, and
that his views now were even more emphatic and extreme "because
time has not proved them erroneous."

CRITICS OF FOCAL INFECTION ARE "LAZY" OR "DISHONEST" [p. 3]
   Fischer asserts as "proved" that a wide range of diseases,
including various internal, nerve, eye and skin diseases, are the
result of embolic infection, and that critics are either "too
lazy mentally" to offer some alternative explanation or "too

dishonest to admit that they do not know".

BILLINGS NECESSITATES REVOLUTION AND "ABOUT FACE" IN MEDICINE [3]
   Fischer characterizes discoveries of the Billings school as
requiring a "revolution" in medical theory and "complete about-
face" in medical practice.

BILLINGS DEFINED THE "DYNAMICS OF PHYSIOLOGICAL PROCESS"
   From 1898, when he assumed the chair of medicine at Rush
Medical College, Billings taught that the circumstances of many
conditions (e.g. lobar pneumonia, meningitis, pleuritis,
arthritis, appendicitis, gall bladder disease, rheumatism,
endocarditis) could only be explained by bacterial infection sown
through the bloodstream. These ideas slowly found their way into
print, e.g. pericarditis in 1901, pernicious anemia correlated
with diseased mouth and teeth in 1902, gastric and duodenal ulcer
in 1906. According to Fischer, "Philosophically, Billings had
replaced the statics of the dead-house by the dynamics of
physiological process."

NEURAL TRANSMISSION DISPUTED [34]
   On the question of whether peripheral (nerve) manifestations of
herpes are secondary to ganglionic effect, Fischer notes that
Rosenow and associates adopted the "sounder point of view ...
[that] the whole clinical picture is the product of a blood-borne
infectious process..."

NERVOUS SYSTEM DISEASES, POLIO, MS, CFS, FROM FOCI [p. 36-7]
   The related pathologies of polio and MS, and other nervous
system diseases, are discussed. Also, mention here and elsewhere
is made of patients who are "tired" without effort or discernible
cause ("chronic fatigue symptom"?)

DEFENDS ROSENOW: HAS ANYONE FOUND ANYTHING ELSE? [p. 43]
   Regarding criticism of Rosenow, for having found streptococci
too constantly in all types of systemic disease, Fischer states,
"Well, has anyone found anything else?"

STREPTOCOCCI INDUCE INFECTION ANYWHERE, AT ANY VELOCITY [44]
   Fischer emphasizes that streptococcal infection can involve
"any and every tissue of the body, at any velocity", and that the
organism is so variable that it may cause equally variable
responses.

MOST (99+%) OF FOCI ARE ORAL [48]
   Fischer relates how Billings had conceded that focal infection
was possible anywhere, but that its most probable site was the
mouth. Fischer emphasized that at least 99% of those with
constitutional diseases were so affected due to infected teeth or
tonsils; one percent or less are from all other sources combined.

SINUS INFECTIONS ARE SECONDARY TO JAW AND TOOTH INFECTIONS [49]

Fischer emphasizes that sinuses are NOT a primary focus, nor are the adnoids; these are secondary to jawbone infections, which are themselves secondary to infected teeth.

ENTIRE DIAGRAM OF PRIMARY FOCI: TONSILS AND TEETH [51]
Fischer repeatedly emphasizes that the "entire diagram" of primary causative foci "narrows down to two points -- *the tonsils and the teeth*." Fischer notes wryly how patients who will readily undergo major internal operations "within their abdomens or pelves, gladly yield their colons even", but will resist giving up an infected tooth or tonsil; remarking nonetheless as to how fortunate it is that these first causes of systemic disease (teeth and tonsils) are so accessible and amenable to surgical correction.

WHY ORAL OPERATIONS MAY WORSEN CONDITION [51]
Fischer cautions, "Proper terminus for the patient is, however, difficult of attainment. Grossest error lies in the non-recognition of obviously infected tonsils, teeth and their surrounding tissues. Whereafter not merely incompetent but inadequate surgical attack makes for cropper. ... A tonsil shaved or the peritonsillar infected lymph channels and inflamed scar tissues not removed, a tooth extracted but its adjacent and similarly affected alveolar bone left standing, too frequently excite constitutional reactions compared with which the signs and symptoms that made the victim a patient were trifling."

EVIDENCE OF RESIDUAL TONSILLAR INFECTION [52]
Evidence of residual tonsillar infection to be "found in stumps, in obviously inflamed lymphatic tissue regrowth, in persistently large neck glands, and in tender and thickened tissues lying below a tonsillectomy scar or its upper or lower regions, and readily discoverable by digital examination of the faucial regions of apparently 'clean' throats."

73% OF TONSILS OPERATIONS ARE UNSUCCESSFUL [52]
Fischer relates data by Rhoads and Dick showing that nearly 3/4 of tonsils operations are unsuccessful (73%) because of incomplete removal, and further that residual tonsillar "stumps" were found to harbor more pathogens per gram than infected tonsils being removed for the first time.

DISEASES CORRELATED WITH TONSILS V.S. TEETH [53]
Various tissues are correlated with tonsils/teeth;
- in young, tonsils: heart disease, rheumatism, chorea;
- in older, teeth: cardiac, arthritic, nerve tissue;
- in adults, tonsils: ulcer, append, rheumatism;
   teeth: arthritis, blood vessel, nervous sys.
Beyond this and when both foci exist in a given individual Fischer adds a "clinical correlation that often proves suggestive: microorganisms find happiest bed in those distant hostelries most like home."

"THE TOOTH IS BONE AND ALIVE [56]
   "John Hunter [Natural History of the Human Teeth, 1778] clearly
and simply declared the teeth so many bones set via the
articulations into two other bones. A tooth in its socket is
classic example of the gliding (arthrodial) joint."

TOOTH NERVE IS A BRANCH OF THE TRIGEMINUS [58]
   Fischer points out that the nerve in the pulp of a tooth is a
branch of the trigeminus nerve in humans. By this measure, a
relation between so-called trigeminal neuralgia and infection of
the tooth's nerve exist nearly by definition. Nonetheless,
except for direct spread of bacterial infection from one branch
to another, transmission would presumably be via the bloodstream.

SEEDS OF TOOTH: CONNECTIVE TISSUE [60]
TOOTH LIKENED TO NAIL-COVERED PHALANX, NOT NAIL [60]
   The seeds of tooth are described as connective tissues
surrounded by blood vessel; outer cells are odontoblastic (hard
capsule over nucleus); the morphogenesis of teeth are likened to
the nail- or hoof-covered phalanx.
   It is noted that this characterization might lend to a degree
of confusion, in that "shoes" are often implanted into hooves of
the likes of horses without ill effect. More specifically,
Fischer equates the hoof or nail with the outside enamel shell of
the tooth.
   This distinction does seem to lie at the philosophical center
of the entire issue, or problem, if you will. The dentistry
position, which would allow for indefinite mechanical
manipulations of the tooth without thought of generalized ill
effect, seems to liken the tooth to a covering that is external
to the skin, like a fingernail. The Fischer/physiological
position equates the tooth with the outside bone of a finger, and
the tooth's enamel with the finger's nail.

JUNCTURE OF TOOTH & JAW IS SYNOVIAL JOINT [62]
   Refers to the juncture of tooth and jaw as "the synovial joint"
between them. Seemingly with every reference to this juncture,
Fischer emphasizes its synovial nature.

TOOTH IS COMPOUND FRACTURE WAITING TO HAPPEN [67]
from Fischer's physiological perspective, teeth with a break in
their enamel are likened to "stumps of a fractured bone which
have penetrated the skin".

HEALTH & THE PRICE OF GOLD [69]
   Discussing the problem of lack of concern by a dental patient
who is not yet affected constitutionally as a result of his
infected teeth, Fischer laments that fixed bridgework may be
regarded by some people ... as better than natural teeth because
gold. [Fischer here invokes derogatory racial stereotypes,
whereas "people from all walks of life" may properly be

inserted.]

SYNOVIAL MEMBRANE SURROUNDS BASE OF TOOTH [62]
In a number of instances Fischer refers to "the synovial membrane" which surrounds the tooth, e.g., p. 62, 72, 78, 79

INFECTED TOOTH IS COMPOUND FRACTURE [71]
Here Fischer likens the onset of infection in a tooth to conversion of a simple fracture into a compound one.

ALL CARIES, ETC., IS OSTEOMYELITIS/OSTEITIS [74]
ALL PYORRHEA, ETC., IS ARTHRITIS/SYNOVITIS [74]
Fischer characterizes as osteomyelitis/osteitis: all caries, dentinitis, cementitis, pulpitis; and as synovitis/arthritis: all pericementitis, alveolitis, pyorrhea

CARIES IS NECROSIS AND INVARIABLY INFECTED [75]
Pathologically caries is "necrosis", and "invariably" infected.

FILLINGS ELIMINATE POSSIBILITY OF TOOTH CAVITY HEALING [75]
Fischer offers that a tooth cavity, if cleaned to good bone, tends to glaze over, but this cannot occur if the tooth is filled.

JOINT OPERATIONS ALWAYS PREDISPOSE TO SECONDARY INFECTION [79]
Fischer points out that surgery on even non-infected articulations carries a high risk of secondary infection, causing orthopedists to exercise great caution so as not to scratch or otherwise injure serous coverings. Unfortunately, specialists in gum disease "have never suffered such qualms."

PULLING TEETH DOES NOT ELIMINATE INFECTION [80]
Jaw infection persists after teeth are pulled.

STREPTOCOCCUS V. OTHER ORAL MICROORGANISMS [81-3]
Fischer refers to numerous microorganisms found in the mouth, frequently in association with systemic diseases, dismissing those whose affects are confined to the mouth (e.g. thrush, amoebae in pyorrhea pockets, and numerous "saprophytes" not also found in distant systemic lesions (micrococci, bacilli, spirochetes).

HEAVY METALS & ORGANISMS PREPARE GROUND FOR STREPTOCOCCUS [81-3]
At the same time Fischer emphasizes possible importance of these organisms in preparing the oral tissue for invasion by the organisms that do have systemic effects. In this connection, Fischer refers to oral manifestations of syphilis, TB, and Vincent's spirillum infection, and likewise to "ground rotted of rickets, scurvy, the HEAVY METAL poisonings, etc.", as fostering conditions for growth of staphylococcus and streptococcus, in all its variations. Fischer once again emphasizes that it is the streptococcus that "is most largely responsible for the

constitutional disasters here under discussion."

MOIST V.S. DRY FORMS OF INFECTION ABOUT TEETH [83-5]
The reaction of infection in and about the teeth is characterized as one of two forms - moist and dry. The moister type when extracted tend to drain more freely and are more apt to involve a clean healing of the jaw state. While the bottom line for both is infection by the same sort of organism, Fischer offers that while the moist form "may be as vivid as a mining camp prostitute, the second is likely to prove as anemic as a New England spinster." For this reason, the latter is too commonly ignored.
Even teeth untouched by dentistry in older persons are a problem, as they tend to involve the dry, "more disastrous" form.

DRY FORM OF TOOTH INFECTION, UNIVERSAL BY AGE 60   [84-5]
According to Fischer, by the time persons have reached 50 or 60 years of age, the dry form of tooth infection is common to the point of being universal." This condition is found primarily in those who had practiced good hygiene, and with what experts might otherwise proclaim perfectly good teeth.

SIGNS OF INFECTION IN TEETH NEVER DENTISTRIED [85]
The following signs in teeth that have never been dentistried are to be critically viewed:
-- polishing off of biting and grinding surfaces to the extent that they expose their dentine and render more vulnerable the pulps;
-- junctional line between tooth and gum showing wear and/or erosion as a result of 3-4 decades of bacterial attack;
-- loss of translucency of tooth crowns, and assumption of whiter, more china-like look;
-- slight recessions of gum with exposure of root substance;
-- firmer fixation of tooth in socket
-- x-ray evidence of possible pulp stones and/or increased calcium deposition in surrounding jawbone.
It is noted that on extraction such a tooth exhibits "a narrowed pulp chamber, with the pulp itself no longer pink and moist but gray and dry with sandy granules sticking in it. (The blood has gone out of it, avascular connective tissue has taken its place and calcium deposit has occurred.)"

EXTRACT TEETH AFTER AGE 60 [86]
Information provided by Fischer seems to be support the position of extraction of all teeth after age 60; see note at bottom [60], referring to the conclusion of Hess and Zürcher in 1925 that by the age of 60 even non-dentistried, normal teeth are affected by a "dry" dentinitis and alveolitis, and their possible constitutional consequences. This is thought to be less a consequence of age, but rather of infection bound to occur with age.

OLD PEOPLE: EXTRACT ALL TEETH; REMOVE ALL "DENTAL RIDGES" [87]
   Fischer asserts that in order to relieve the old of their
chronic disease symptoms, they need not only have all their
remaining teeth extracted, but must also sacrifice the "dental
ridge" that dentists are inclined to retain for the purpose of
holding dentures better.

NEARLY EVERYTHING IN DENTISTRY IS WRONG [90]
ALL FILLINGS MUST GO; WRONG IN PRINCIPLE [90]
   Fischer asserts that nearly everything in dentistry is wrong is
principle and must be stopped, including all fillings:
   "In our opinion, nearly everything he [the dentist] is doing
is wrong, for it turns out that with scarce an exception everyone
of the tooth-saving devices that he has engendered is wrong in
principle. 'they must in consequence be given up. It means that
the following are of the past: all his dental de-vitalizations,
root canal fillings, pivot teeth, root amputations, fixed
bridges, crowns, larger inlays, tooth straightening procedures
employing such schemes, too rapid movements of the teeth (in
orthodontic practice or in tooth wedgings to get at inter-dental
lesions), undercut fillings, other kinds if large; and finally --
it must be said softly -- all fillings."

"PESSIMISTIC CONCLUSION [90-1]
   Fischer goes on to discuss other problem practices in
dentistry, e.g., "picky" tools, incomplete eradication of
infection, undercutting, use of cements to retain fillings, etc.,
concluding pessimistically:
   "can [the dentist] do enough by anything short of extraction
to eradicate a locus of infection? Examination of any carious
tooth in cross section will give pause, for bacteria have usually
penetrated far beyond the limits of his cutting."[91]

ALL PULPLESS TEETH ARE BAD, HOWEVER "WELL" FILLED [94-5]
   Fischer relates the conclusions of a number of dentists and
others who found that all pulpless teeth are bad, and that there
is no difference in the result whether the teeth are properly
filled or not at all.

PATIENT MUST CLEAN OWN TEETH; DENTIST CAN'T DO IT [99]
   Fischer cites Hartzell (former ADA President) as having
asserted: "If a patient cannot clean his own teeth, no dentist
can do it for him."

DANGERS OF TOOTH CLEANING [101]
   If a tooth is scaled below the gum line, at best the dentist is
killing a synovial membrane and at worst helping to diffuse an
infection aiming to do the same. Results, if the patient does
not die, are synovial tissue death, hastened gum retraction,
cementum death, ankylosis.

VIRTUALLY EVERYTHING IN DENSTISTRY IS WORTHLESS AND DANGEROUS

[102]

Fischer concludes that everything in dentistry (except very early, very superficial things and extractions) is at once "useless and dangerous."

FAILURE OF MEDICINE AND DENTISTRY FEEDS ALTERNATIVE APPROACHES
[107]

Fischer blames medicine and dentistry's failure to properly deal with focal diseases for contributing to the numbers of patients who desperately seek out the likes of barbers, cosmeticians, masseurs, colon irrigators, chiropractors, Christian sciencers, drug clerks, physical therapists and other alternative medical practitioners:

"Whenever our professions assume that a 'naturally progressive' disease must remain such, or that help for the patient lies beyond medical understanding and surgical help, it contributes membership to that easy third of the chronically ill which in desperation becomes the clientele of bargers, cosmeticians, masseurs, colon irrigators, chiropractors, osteopaths, and Christian sciencers. It is the point of view that has turned over to drug clerks with their pain killers and to physical therapists with their machinery, no small fraction of a public that originally sought medical council."

DIFFICULTY IN FINDING FOCI [107-8]

Fischer quotes Rosenow on the difficulty of revealing the identity of harmful foci:
"The place of entrance of these organisms is often difficult to determine. The associated tonsillitis in rheumatism when an attack comes on is nearly always mild, while in chronic infectious endocarditis there is often no apparent tonsillitis or one which is [108] no more marked than in many normal individuals. ... It is safe to say that the focus is most commonly found in the oral cavity and here the order of frequency is the tonsil, pyorrhea and blind abscesses about the teeth."

Fisher relates that Rosenow had to ignore the inability of specialists to find foci, equipping himself with specialists' equipment and getting infectious material out of tonsils and gums that the experts had declared uninfected. "(More history to show that specialists never make basic contribution to their specialty -- *rank outsiders are needed*".)

"CLINICAL HUNT FOR DENTAL AND PERIDENTAL INFECTION" [109]

Fischer carries on for a half-dozen pages on how to go about poking in the various nooks and crannies in the mouth for typical "focal infections". He notes that x-ray examination does not reveal early changes in soft tissues, nor spread of infection, nor does it necessarily reveal changes in shade due to calcium variations. The plusses of x-rays are then discussed, but with the qualification that the physical exam is more important.

PHYSICAL EXAM. OF TEETH [110-111]

Discoloration is equated with deprivation of blood supply and death; loss of transparency is equated with increased, abnormal calcium deposition. Areas of caries, fillings, crowns or pegged teeth that smell foully "are self labeled"; areas that are hyper or hypo sensitive are all infected; as are red, swollen or bleeding gums, structures sensitive to finger ball pressure, pus or scummy white line about the tooth neck.

LIVE TOOTH CAN BE FOCUS [111]
   Fischer bemoans "a popular type of ignorance" that argues that a tooth cannot be infected because it is alive, which he equates with saying that a patient cannot have a carbuncle on his neck "because he is still breathing."

TONSILS: BEWARE OF SHRUNKEN, RIND-LIKE, "NORMALLY ATROPHIC" [111]
   Fischer urges awareness of tonsils that are "shrunken and made rind-like" and often thought of as "normally atrophic".

THINGS TO LOOK FOR IN TEETH, SIGNS OF INFECTION [112]
a. gum recession
b. discoloration about neck or biting edge
c. erosion
d. loss of transparency

The importance of the above mounts with:
e. teeth that are unduly fast
f. unduly loose
g. laterally placed fillings, especially if beneath the gum line
h. encroachment of dentine upon pulp chamber
i. pulp stones.

Fischer emphasizes that "we have never failed to recover partial tension microorganisms from structures so affected."

INFECTION IN JAWBONE AS IMPORTANT AS IN TOOTH [112]
   Fischer considers it "self-evident" that residual jawbone infections are as important as infected teeth or gums in terms of serving as possible seeding foci. He bemoans that the former has received very little consideration, and this in turn has caused people to condemn extractions on the grounds that they do no good. Says Fischer: *"Still active nidi of infection were left in the jaw and nothing adequate was done about them."*

INFECTION IN NON-DENTISTRIED TEETH [112; see also 85-6]
   Signs of infection in older persons without dentistry are reiterated.

LACK OF PAIN, ETC. IS THE RULE IN ORAL FOCI [113-114]
   Fischer discusses in turn how each group of oral foci was pretty-much painless, but nonetheless deadly. While pain in or around a tooth is a sure sign of infection, the infected tooth generally does not hurt, nor does the infected tonsil. Mention

of the synoviae and jawbone, in this connection, are also discussed, with the notation that in order to produce pain, an infection must induce swelling in some structure within the dento-alveolar joint area.

HEAVY METAL POISONING PREDISPOSES TO INFECTION [114]
Interestingly, Fischer points out that metallic poisoning or scurvy can cause the same type of pain, and further that such chemically affected tissues are found to become infected not long afterwards.
This might help explain why mercury toxicity in teeth correlates so well with diseases that Rosenow et al. had shown to be caused by infection; the presence of such toxic substances does, according to Fischer, encourage the presence of infection.

TONSILS, BEWARE OF SMALL, FIRM, WITH GREEN PUS ON PRESSURE [114]
Watch for tonsils that are smaller and firmer than normal, from which a greenish pus is expressible on pressure.

EXTRACTION OF NON-DENTISTRIED TEETH MOST IMPORTANT [115]
Recounting all the failed dental practices and need to render extinct all "these surgical leftovers", Fischer then emphasizes that it is more important to recognize and extract "equally affected teeth" that have never been touched by dentistry but nonetheless are an important source of infection to the body in general.

NEED TO EXTRACT RESIDUALLY-INFECTED JAWBONE [120]
Fischer discusses in depth the need to extract residually-infected peridental bone.

MUTUAL INTERDEPENDENCE OF TEETH AND JAW PER J. HUNTER [120]
Fischer quotes John Hunter, *A Practical Treatise on the diseases of the Teeth*, 7, J. Johnson, London (1778): "... there is such mutual dependence of the teeth, and alveolar processes on each other, that the destruction of the one seems to be always attended with that of the other."

JAWBONE OPERATION SOMETIMES POSTPONED MONTH OR TWO [120]
"We do not always dress to the ultimate resorption line at once, simply because the alveolar bone is infected and line of demarcation of infection is 'vague'. ... for a month or two after an extraction we incline to let the patient rest, in order better to know how much of what remains of peridental bone assumes healthy form. Then the still affected alveolar process, now more definitely demarcated, is attacked a second time."

SURE SIGNS OF INFECTION [121]
- every area of gum that is still reddened, and every area that is sensitive to finger ball pressure, indicates an area of infection underneath

EVERY EXTRACTION IS GREEN STICK, COMPOUND, FRACTURE [121]
According to Fischer, every "ordinary" extraction is a compound "comminuted or green stick fracture" and must be treated accordingly.

GENERAL ANESTHETICS PREFERRED OVER LOCAL [122]
Fischer points out that local anesthetics do not benefit pathologically affected tissues, and recommends general anesthesia as better suited for oral surgery.

ANESTHESIA DANGER [123]
Fischer warns that anesthetics make tissues, including nerve tissue swell, and cautions that an anesthetized dental nerve within its canal "may strangle itself".

ALCOHOL PRIOR TO INJECTING NOVOCAINE, & FOR PAIN [125]
In that the antidote of cocaine and derivatives is alcohol, Fischer employs no morphine or its derivates, and never atropine. Brandy or whiskey is administered, an ounce or two a few minutes before injection of novocaine and another ounce or two after the operation. Alcohol is also advocated to ameliorate post-op pain in days following.

CALL FOR CAREFUL AFTER-TREATMENT [126]
Fischer equates after-treatment of an extraction site as at best that of a fracture and compound; or worse, a pathological situation -- osteomyelitis, periostitis, osteitis.

AUTOTHERAPY [127]
Fischer discusses reasons for beneficial action of saliva on a wound, building on the knowledge of beneficial effects of animals licking their wounds. The beneficial action of saliva is partly attributed to the existence of a concentration of several salts.

IRRIGATING SOLUTIONS [128-9]
For an irrigating solution, Fischer recommends strong and hot salt water, strong enough, hot enough and long enough, with concentration never below one percent; two to five percent is better. For quick preparation, a level teaspoonful (4 gm) of table salt is dissolved in a glass (150cc) of hot water. Fischer prefers mixed salts as described below.
In freshly operated osteomyelitic foci, even a 1 or 2 percent NaCl solution may not be adequate.

IRRIGATING SOLUTION - RECIPE [130]
Fischer's recommended dressing or irrigant for routine surgical use:

NaCl	10.5
CaCl (dried)	0.84
KCl	0.42
Distilled H2O (enough to make)	1000.00

(note: dissolve CaCl and KCl first, and then add NaCl.)

Fischer discusses irrigation solutions in greater detail on p. 130-132.

IMPORTANCE OF REMOVAL OF SYNOVIAE AND BONE [136]
  As he had previously emphasized on p. 120 and earlier, Fischer emphasizes that failure to adequately remove surrounding infection at the time of extraction will become a problem in the future.

NEED TO BE AGGRESSIVE IN BONE SURGERY [136]
  Fischer asserts that the surgeon must go down at least to "'true' bone constituting the maxillae proper." He advocates removing saved periosteum, as this has invariably necessitated a second operation for its removal.

REMOVE PETROUS WALLS AND ROUND OFF MEDULLARY [137]
  Bone removal - remove petrous walls first, rounding off medullary portion, as in fig. 43 facing p. 87

"SAVING" INFECTED JAW BONE IS DEBIT IN BOOK OF LIFE [137]
  "Every attempt to "save" [infected jaw-]bone ... enters debits upon the book of life ... ." Fischer emphasizes that he had not seen a single patient die of a focal-origin disease who, despite having had all teeth removed (and proper tonsillectomy) did not have residual infection in the jaws.

LACK OF EXTRACTION BENEFIT DUE TO RESIDUAL INFECTION [137]
  As elsewhere, Fischer scoffs at the argument commonly cited as "proof" against the focal infection concept, i.e., that patients who have had multiple or total extractions had not been constitutionally benefited, retorting, "these patients were never properly freed by surgical method of their first foci!"

CLOTS, EXTRACTION POCKETS; FISCHER ADVOCATES EARLY REMOVAL OF [138]
  Fischer offers that 'formation of a clot'" in spaces from which teeth have been extracted is not necessarily good, except that it shows that circulation to the place was good. "The clots that form in extraction pockets require the earliest possible, and continuous, removal.
  "The 'good' of which bleeding into a socket speaks, is a maintained blood supply."

DISASTROUS EFFECTS OF ONE BAD TOOTH IN 16 YEAR OLD [143]
  Effects of one bad tooth on 16-year-old high school boy are discussed.

RHEUMATISM IMPROVED FOLLOWING EXTRACTION [145]
  Chronic rheumatism, including all the joints of both hands and feet, in a 23-year-old woman; condition improved following extraction of infected teeth.

INFECTION, EDENTULOUS JAWS [146]
   Fischer emphasizes and illustrates how edentulous jaws are not necessarily, or even rarely, free from infection.

RHEUMATOID ARTHRITIS IMPROVED WHEN RIDGE GROUND OFF [146-7]
   Discusses a case where rheumatic conditions affected joints of fingers, knee joint, and ankle; the rheumatic conditions subsided when the alveolar ridge was ground off.
   This patient was already edentulous but could not work as sculptress due to pain in hands, knuckles showing a thickening and sensitiveness and there was difficulty in bending or extending fingers. There was also swelling about right knee and ankle joints causing limp.
   Fischer laments that a first operation, in which 5 socket areas in the lower left jaw were laid open and curetted, had not been sufficiently radical. "The gum should have been split and all the serrations flattened to smooth line by slow moving burr with this dressing of the jaw bone directed as per the curved line inked into Figure 43." (opposite p. 87) From three days after the necessary, second, jawbone operation, the patient was well.

CARDIAC PROBLEMS ETC, CURED WHEN IMPLICATED TEETH EXTRACTED [148]
   50 year-old female physician, in bed for a year, blue-lipped when flat, cyanotic and dyspneic when she tried to rise; with cardiac & problems, etc., was cured when her (20) implicated teeth were extracted.

BREAST TUMOR DISAPPEARED AFTER EXTRACTIONS [148-9]
   50 year old female patient with very tender tumor in her left breast, under the edge of the areola. The tumor disappeared after infected teeth were properly removed. Fischer related that he had long thought that such a tumor, discovered due to its tenderness, is probably of inflammatory origin.
   Fischer relates having had similar experiences in several women, with diagnosis of tumor corrected to diagnosis of metastatically induced mastitis.

BREAST LUMP DISAPPEARED AFTER MOLARS EXTRACTED [150]
   40 year old farmer's wife, with walnut-sized lump in lower, outer quadrant of left breast, sensitive, involving two thickened and tender ducts, disappeared following gradual removal of 5 molars.

PATIENT REFUSES JAW SURGERY, DIES [151-2]
   Here patient is discussed who had sugar in urine, heightened blood pressure, swollen testicles (metastatic origin). Tonsils and teeth were removed, but subsequent distress in left chest and arm, edema in feet ascending into liver and abdomen. Edentulous jaws were still serrated, red and tender on pressure, but refused surgery. Died, at age 59, within two months of onset of chest and arm pain.

ARTHRITIS, GASTRIC, EYE PROBLEMS YIELD TO JAW OPERATION [152]
   45 year old housewife, tired all the time, hands tended to
swell, gastric, gall bladder and eye problems all cleared after
remains of infected alveolar processes were ground off.

IDENTICAL ETIOLOGY OF WIDELY SPACED SYSTEMIC DISEASES [155]
   Emphasizes that the physician must recognize that identical
etiology and pathology underlie systemic diseases that may be
widely spaced both in location in the body and years, terming
these all parts of the "Billings-Rosenow syndrome".

VARIOUS DISEASES CORRELATED WITH ORAL FOCI [156ff]
   Following is a brief recounting of some of the disease
conditions discussed by Fischer in his case studies section,
which call for the surgical removal of oral foci (infected
tonsils, teeth or jawbone):
   -- recurrent or long persistent vesicular, pustular, crusting
and sclerosing forms of irregularly distributed skin eruption;
   -- dendritic keratitis
   -- allergy
   -- eye diseases
   -- nephritis
   -- rheumatism of hand joints
   -- cystitides and prostatitides
   -- pain in bladder region
   -- enlargement of prostate
   -- patchy types of nervous system disease
   -- various non-inherited manifestations of pancreas, thyroid,
pituitary, suprarenal, gonadal, diseases, including e.g.
impotence; and more.

RHEUMATOID ARTHRITIS DISAPPEARS WHEN JAW RIDGES CUT AWAY [161]
   Patient (woman) had rheumatism which had thickened all the
joints of her hands. Attacks did not permanently disappear until
jaw ridges were cut away.

BLADDER SYMPTOMS IMPROVE AFTER JAWS ROUNDED [162-3]
   Patient with bladder symptoms that improved with pulling of bad
teeth did not fully improve until tender areas in jaws were
removed and jaws had healed to rounded and smooth arches.

ALKALINITY ENCOURAGED [163]
   Fischer describes keeping urine alkaline with fruit juice,
vegetable diet, and sodium bicarbonate and magnesium and calcium
carbonate, during the period when extractions are occurring; but
emphasizes the true benefits were a result of the extractions
themselves.

AUTONOMIC NERVOUS SYSTEM DAMAGE, NERVOUS SYSTEM DISEASE, CAUSED
BY BACTERIAL INFECTION [164]
   Fischer discusses the role of bacterial infection emanating
from oral foci as cause of autonomic nervous system damage and

nervous system disease.

POST-POLIO, CHRONIC FATIGUE, OTHER NERVOUS DISEASES [166]
Fischer refers to hard-to-classify patients with various different combinations of symptoms and are "tired all the time".

Reference is also made to various nervous system maladies not thought of as chronic focal infection diseases, which should be, including post meningitic, post-poliomyelitic, post influenzal, post-pneumococcic, and post-streptococcic.

TRIGEMINAL NEURALGIA, FACIAL TICS DUE TO INFECTED TEETH [169]
Fischer asserts that trifacial neuralgias, facial tics, and overall, "primary infection in the migrainous lies most commonly in their teeth."

HEADACHES IN EDENTULOUS CURED WHEN SERRATED JAW BURRED OFF [171]
Patient had suffered various constitutional symptoms, particularly headaches, until edentulous jaws were opened and remaining serrations burred off. Only then was he able to return to work.

RHEUMATIC PAINS, HEMMORHOIDS RELIEVED AFTER JAW OP. [173]
Woman with hemmorhoids and rheumatic pains, who had earlier had varicose veins treated by injection, with heat and edema in leg, and area of near necrosis over the malleolus, was freed of all constitutional symptoms ("except her dilated and tortuous veins") only after losing all remaining exostotic and tender alveolar processes.

INITIAL INSULT IS CAPILLARY IN NATURE [176]
Discusses Gull and Sutton's concept of arterio-capillary-venous fibrosis, whereby initial insult is capillary in nature.

EXCESSIVE CHOLESTEROL NOT DISEASE CAUSE [177]
Fischer points out that the cholesterol fed guinea pigs by Anitschkow, and subsequently verified, had produced a lipoidemia, wherein floating fat particles acted as so many emboli. However to get this effect, the animals were given for 127 days the equivalent of 40 eggs per day, concluding that this does not justify the assumption that excessive consumption of cholesterol in man is related to disease.

HEADACHE & BLINDNESS RELIEVED AFTER JAWBONE BURRED OFF [181-3]
patient with left-sided headache and blindness was only relieved of symptoms after residual infections in jaw were burred off.

CHRONIC SINUS DISEASE SECONDARY TO ORAL INFECTION [187]
Relates that chronic sinus disease "often in our observations proved to be extension effect merely from mouth infection."

BOIL ON SKIN ANALOGOUS TO BOIL ON PANCREAS, IN DIABETES [189]

Fischer injects reference to the "historic association of superficial boils with diabetes." Fischer suggests the "boil" on the skin are merely the analogue of a "boil" in the pancreas, and both from the same source.

Reimann 1940 ARTICLE EQUATED WITH STUPIDITY [198]
   Fischer refers to ignorant actions of the past, then to Reimann's 1940 JAMA article in terms of: "These stupidities are not yet come to an end." [Note that this Reimann article (a) was wholly dependent on Holman's fraudulent 1928 handiwork for refutation of Rosenow's work; and (b) came to serve as the key citation in Beeson's landmark 1976 Bi-Centennial rejection of the focal infection concept.]

RUSH COMBINED REMOVAL OF FOCUS WITH AUTOHEMOTHERAPY (I.E. BLOODLETTING) [199]
   The work of Benjamin Rush is discussed, involving oral focus removal followed by a small quantity of bloodletting.

GOUT RELATED TO TEETH [202]

FUTILITY OF FURTHER SPECIALIZATION IN MEDICINE [209]
   Cautions against further specialization in medicine, "because the individual cannot be split... .

TONSILS AND TEETH ARE NESTS FOR DISEASE; NOWHERE ELSE [210]
   "... it is almost exclusively in the tonsils and in the teeth that the infectious microorganisms responsible for constitutional disease find permanent lodging -- and not anywhere else!"

TOOTH BUDS FORMED BY 4TH MONTH [211]
   Tooth buds - signs of growth and calcification are seen as early as 4th month. [Thus it may be speculated that from such a point in time might be calculated the time required to grow (e.g. clone) new teeth.

MILK IS LIQUID TISSUE [212]
   "Milk is the broken down tissue of the mother herself."

"RACKETEERING" IN JAMA [215]
   Fischer offhandedly characterizes food supplement advertising in JAMA as "racketeering", emphasizing that of greater importance is their chemical composition; Fischer asserted that the proper proportion and quality are found in raw animal foodstuffs.

DRINK WITH MEALS BAD FOR TEETH [219]
   Fischer asserts that drinking with meals is very bad for the teeth, not for the stomach as is more commonly assumed. The drinking with the meals keeps the teeth from cleaning themselves by mastication.

PURPOSE OF DENTIFRICE IS DEHYDRATION [220]

Dentifrice: NaCl solution better than water; alkaline salt better yet, e.g. baking soda; or for more abrasion, $CaCO_3$ or $MgCO_3$, or oxide or hydroxide; permit time to soak into tissues of mouth.

"NONSENSE", THE FILLING OF TEETH IS [221-2]

Tooth fillings are "nonsense. Would the state of an osteomalacic bone be improved by having some lead bullets -- even if sterile -- pounded into it?"

INFECTED TEETH - THE LESS DONE THE BETTER [223]

Fischer recommends that at most an obviously infected tooth should be burred off, and if the entrance is narrow and fans out, it should be widened. Beyond this he suggests bathing with strong salt water, alkaline dentifrices, and applying tincture of iodine, which measures have seemed to be of benefit. but it should never be closed off or filled.

BONE SPICULES FROM HYPODERMIC ANESTHESIA AND MYOSITIS [223]

Fischer links bone spicules, which may follow the tracks of previous hypodermic injection of anesthetics, to "the ossificans half of myositis".

REIMANN RIDICULED BY ROSENOW [225]

Refers to Rosenow taking a crack back at Reimann (Arch. Int. Med. 62, 602), in response to Reimann's having criticized Rosenow for having found so many diseases as linked to the streptococcus. Rosenow noted that Reimann missed four.

CHRONIC FATIGUE SYNDROME [226]

Refers to those chronically fatigued, but who do not fit into any typical diagnostic category. Fischer aptly notes that saving the patient is as important as saving the tooth.

OKELL AND ELLIOTT SEEN AS SUPPORTING FOCAL INFECTION [228]

Fischer refers to Okell and Elliott (whose results Grossman, in several editions of his Root-Canal/Endodontics textbooks, had twisted to suit his own purposes) as having "noted a streptococus viridans bacteremia in sixty-one percent of 138 patients immediately after extraction with the 'amount of damage done' at operation held responsible for their highest counts." Fischer regarded such bacteriemias to not contraindicate operations, but rather to properly prepare the patient and use gentle surgical technic.

DOCTORS V.S. DENTISTS; EDUCATED V.S. TECHNICAL [229]

Fischer refers to a stalemate between educated doctors without technical skills, on the one hand, versus technicians (dentists) without education.

DENTISTRY REFERRRED TO AS ABORTION [229]

Fischer refers to the first institution in 1840 that was

devoted to training in dentistry as "devoted to nurture of the abortion".

EXTRACTION IS NOT FOR BOY SCOUTS [230]
  "Tooth pulling is no longer boy scout first aid ... "

ONLY (ORAL) INFECTION IS RESPONSIBLE FOR CHRONIC DISEASES [231]
    Fischer final paragraph asks the rhetorical question as to whether "only infection is responsible for" a long list of diseases, eleven lines-worth of a list, concluding with "That, Gentlemen, is exactly what we mean."

    * * * * * *

Addendum 1 to Review of Fischer's Death and Dentistry:

Supplementary Index to Death and Dentistry
    Following is an index of terms/items discussed above. This
index is supplementary to the index published in the original
work; above-discussed items are incorporated below both as line
items and within topical groupings:

     * * * * * *

Addendum 2 to Review of Fischer's Death and Dentistry:
Items of interest from predecessor articles cited on p. 232,
Death & Dentistry:

A. Martin H. Fischer, *Dental Summary*, August 1915, Vol. 35, 607,
from an address to the Cincinnati Dental Society, Jan. 29, 1915,
613-622, 716-734:
   DEVITALIZATION OF TOOTH [719]
   "To devitalize means, of course, to rob a tooth of its life,
and yet when I have discussed this question with dentists they
are likely to talk about the procedure as if it meant a mere
robbing of the tooth of its nerve supply. There is a fundamental
error in this view. ... he simultaneously robs it of its
central, nutrient artery ... . This destruction of the central
blood supply to the tooth is analogous to the cutting off of the
nutrient artery to one of the long bones, the inevitable result
of which is a death of the bone marrow."... [719]
   "Whether we call the dead bone a dead root or a devitalized
tooth or what you will, the problem is exactly the same. We need
to get rid of these as of dead bone elsewhere in the body, and
then the infection will usually take care of itself." [725]
   "... if a certain procedure is wrong in principle when invoked
for surgical purposes anywhere in the body, it must be equally
wrong when the attempt is made to fit it to the special problem
of the teeth.
[732]

B. Martin Fischer, "Some Physiologic Principles in Orthodontia",
International Journal of Orthodontia and Oral Surgery, Vol. 9,
1923, 16-30:
   "Every type of filling, either root canal fillings, temporary
gutta percha fillings or permanent met al. fillings, are to be
avoided. By sealing away organisms in the absence of oxygen all
these procedures become dangerous." [24]
   "Denial of existence of infection by a dentist does not mean
that none is present." [30]

C. M.H. Fischer, "Edema", in Piersol, G.M., *Cyclopedia of
Medicine*, 1939:
   ALKALOSIS SCARCELY EXISTS
"Even with the chemical disposition in volatile form of any
alkali introduced into or produced in the body declared
impossible, there is always plenty of acid available to
neutralize all but colossal doses of such alkali. In the case of
the human being, for example, the amount of carbonic acid
produced daily is sufficient to neutralize 2 pounds of caustic
soda and such doses of alkali are scarcely to be anticipated even
in cases of alkali poisoning. ('Alkalosis', meaning by the term
-- 'poisoning with alkali' ... -- therefore scarcely exists
clinically. What is termed such is an intoxication with light
metals, particularly K and Na.)"

Section 6. The Legend of the Toothworm, 5000 BC - 2000 AD

As we enter a new millennium, it is clear from a review of the dental pre-history up through the present time that the world of dental practice is still firmly in the grasp of the venerable legend of the tooth worm. Supposedly we, the civilized ones of the late 20th and early 21st centuries, are past such nonsense, with only isolated uncivilized "vulgar" peoples still in its grasp. Wrong.

The concept of emptying the contents of an infected tooth, as prominently practiced (indeed, the centerpiece, culmination, guiding and enabling principle of progressive intervention) in contemporary dentistry cannot be reconciled with the modern and indisputable physiological knowledge that the tooth is basically a bone. But this practice of emptying out the central canal(s) of the tooth makes perfect sense within the context of the tooth worm.

Even in modern times, an extirpated pulp may be dangled (as though it is a worm) before the patient, who may be cautioned not to touch this dangerously infected thing. If the patient were to be informed that this is the bone marrow, and that a soon-to-be dead and grossly infected bone has been and will be left sticking out of the skin, would this be tolerated?

It is clear that "root-canal-therapy" generally stops the pain in toothache. However, it does this by removing the tooth's central nerve (along with nutrient-providing circulation, etc.), which nerve is the very source of pain within the tooth. But it does not cure the tooth, it does not remove all infection from the tooth, it does not assure the future sterility of the tooth, and it does nothing to forestall or prevent systemic diseases that are known to come from oral foci. The inescapable conclusion to be drawn from perhaps 7000 years of history is that so-called "root-canal-therapy" is the absurdly bogus modern attempt to vanquish the tooth worm -- this with a modern "spin" on the operation so as to make it sound like something scientifically beneficial is being accomplished.

Thus it is clear that the tooth worm will not be vanquished until so called "root canal therapy" and even all of tooth carpentry is vanquished (except for some yet-to-be-discovered truly-curative form is devised).

Following are a number of versions of translations of the ancient Sumerian writings describing the cause of toothache, followed by various accounts of the tooth worm through the pre-history of dentistry:

A. Translations of the Legend of the Toothworm:

It is noted that slightly different twists are taken in the various translations of this legend, particularly in the parts in which the worm speaks. On may surmise that by reading all of these accounts, one may gain a better understanding of the nuances of the original writer, in that we do not otherwise have a precise bona fide verifiable single translation.

The timing of the original formulation of the tooth worm hypothesis is generally thought to be about 5000 BC. For example, Christine Hillam, Ed., Roots of Dentistry, Brit. Dent. J., 1990, p. 55 states that a Sumerian clay tablet from 5000 BC described worms as the cause of caries and gave remedies for toothache. There may be some confusion in that the ancient Tablet describing this legend may have been found within a collection of materials from a library from about 3000 BC, which may be why some authors refer this as 5000 year old material. Rather than quibble about a mere couple of millennia, we will accept that the tooth worm concept is at least 5000-7000 years old.

With our limited life span and far more limited attention span, it is useful to reflect momentarily on a civilization of 5000-7000 years ago that had preserved records and passed them intact to modern times. The wisdom underlying this tremendous feat of preservation seems to provide a stark contrast to modern destructive tendencies, whereby a relatively young militaristic society is capable of inflicting horrendous physical destruction on a traditional society thousands of miles distant with relative impunity. This is of particular interest in the current political milieu when it is realized that the birthplace of civilization as we know it, this grand Sumerian tradition, is the delta area of the Tigris and Euphrates rivers, in an area now known as Iraq. One wonders what, if anything, will be left of the record we are now creating 5000-7000 years hence.

And of the tooth itself, so little practical knowledge has been gained in the past 5000-7000 years that one must wonder how much will be gained in the next. How long will it take to learn how to banish tooth infections, and what will be the implications for the lifespan of human beings? We are well in the era of the century-long lifespan, and may have been here for quite a while.
 How long before the two-century lifespan? By then will we have learned how to turn the clock back for a time, so that it can be run forward again, and how long before these doubling exercises will yield the millennium-long lifespan?

1. Leo Kanner, Folklore of the Teeth, MacMillan, NY, 1928, p. 107.

After Anu (had created the heavens),
The heavens created the earth,
The earth created the rivers,
The rivers created the canals,
The canals created the marsh,
The marsh created the worm,
Then came the worm weeping before Shamash;
Before Ea came her tears:

"What wilt thou give me for my food?
What wilt thou give me as mine to destroy?"

"I will give thee the ripe figs and soft pomegranates."

"Me! What are these ripe figs to me, and soft pomegranates?
Lift me up, between the teeth and the jaw-bone set me,
That I may destroy the blood of the teeth,
And ruin their strength,
Grasp the prong and seize the root."

2. R.C. Thompson, London, per Prinz, Dental Chronology, Lea &
Febiger, Phila., 1945: "About 5000 BC.: Legend of the Worm

"After Anu (had created the Heavens) the Heavens created (the
Earth), the Earth created the Marshes, the Marshes created the
Worm. Came the Worm (and) wept before Shamash, before Ea came
his tears:

'What wilt thou give me for my food, what wilt thou give me for
my devouring?'

'I will give thee dried bones, (and) scented -wood.'

'What are these dried bones to me, and scented ... -wood' 'Let
me drink among the teeth, and set me on the gums; that I may
devour the blood of the teeth and of their gums destroy the
strength; then shall I hold the bolt of the door.'

'So must thou say this: O Worm. May Ea smite thee with the might
of his fist!' 'Thus shalt pulverize henbane and knead it with
gum mastic and place it in the upper part of the tooth, and three
times shalt recite this incantation.'"

3. Lillian Lindsay, Short History of Dentistry, Bale & Sons,
London 1933, p. 8, Babylonian texts 3000 BC, on Bricks in the
British Museum:

"The worm or enemy says

'Set me amid the teeth and let me dwell in the gums that I may
destroy the blood of the teeth and of the gums chew their marrow.
 The door is the flesh, the latch is the bone, she hath entered
the flesh, she hath lifted the bone, she hath bitten the flesh,
she hath dug into the bone."

4. The Worm and the Toothache [At Creighton] Translated by E.
A. Speiser, Ancient Near Eastern Texts Related to the Old
Testament, edited by J. B. Pritchard (Princeton: Princeton
University Press, 1969), 100-101.
[Source - WWW: * Britannica - 1 History, 2 Middle East, 3
Ancient Middle East, Level 4 + Sumeria ... --

http://nw1.newsweek.com/nw-srv/inetguide/iguide_4412328.html]

After Anu had created heaven,
Heaven had created the earth,
The earth had created the rivers,
The rivers had created the marsh,
And the marsh had created the worm---
The worm went, weeping, before Shamash,
His tears flowing before Ea:

"What will you give me for food?
What will you give me to suck on?"

"I will give you the ripe fig and the apricot."

"What good is the ripe fig and the apricot?
Lift me up, and assign me to the teeth and the gums!
I will suck the blood of the tooth,
and I will gnaw its roots at the gum!"

"Because you have said this, O worm,
May Ea strike you with the might of his hand!"

B.   Further discussions of and references to the tooth worm
through history. There are some variations in interpretations;
rather than attempting to sort them out, these are presented as
stated by their authors. All in all, the picture painted is that
of a very pervasive role for the tooth worm:

1.   Kanner (Folklore of the Teeth, MacMillan, NY, 1928, 107ff)
provides a rundown of other historical references to the worm:

-- Throughout the middle ages the worm etiology of toothache was
considered scientific fact
-- Gypsy women of India were noted for charms to take out
toothworms
-- In Arabia there were those "who fetch the worm from the tooth
-- Chinese dentists would induce a cough which was intended to
make the worm fall out.
-- In Madagascar toothache sufferers were referred to as "marary
olitra", or "poorly through the worm"
-- Algonkian Indians referred to "mosewabite", a worm in the
tooth
-- In European countries, uneducated people were said to believe
in the worm etiology, as a result of seeing a pulp hanging down
from the root of a carious or broken extracted tooth, which looks
like a worm
-- Orkney Islands inhabitants call toothache "the worm"
-- Isle of Man inhabitants refer to toothache as the plural form
of beast, beishtyn, thinking the pain to come from an animal in
the teeth
-- In Gaelic, cnuimh, a worm, gives rise to the name for

toothache, cnuimh fhiacall
-- Kanner refers to Philip Massinger's "Parliament of Love",
which blames the worm for both toothache and love; and
Shakespeare's "Much Ado About Nothing": Non Pedro: "What! Sigh
for the toothache?" Leonato: "Where is but humour, or a worm."

2. M. D. K. Bremner, DDS, FACD, in discussions of 17th century
dentistry, notes that toothache was commonly attributed to worms,
thinking that breaking open an extracted tooth would allow one to
see the worms. "Dental patients of today also frequently mistake
the pulp for a worm." [The Story of Dentistry, Rev. 3rd Ed.,
Dental Items of Interest Publ. Co., Brooklyn 1954, p. 90-91]

3. W.D. Miller recounts a number of prominent historical
references to the worm theory of caries, mentioning Scribonius,
Ebn-Sina, Musitanus (1114), Kräutermann (1732), Ringelmann
(1824), Kremler and others, who followed Ebn-Sina in recommending
seeds of hanbane, leek and onions or similar measures. Miller
attributes to then-contemporary Chinese dentists the use of an
instrument with a hollow handle containing artificial worms,
which are dropped into the mouth in the middle of an operation
and exhibited as evidence. Miller relates the Japanese term for
toothache as mushi (worm) ba (tooth), and attributes the same
worm-related meaning to the Chinese word for hollow tooth, chung
choo.
    "We must rid ourselves of the impression ... that the
parasites of the human mouth make holes in the dentine by boring
into it as a worm bores into wood.... Bacteria have no apparatus
for boring.... They nourish themselves alone by substances in a
state of solution.... [p. 211]
    Miller notes that Hollarius had questioned the worm theory as
early as 600. [p. 128]
    (Miller also cites Hippocrates as having discussed the
relation of teeth and severe diseases of jaw, and having said,
"The jaw of the son of Metrodorus mortified in consequence of
toothache, and the gums became intensely swollen; the suppuration
was moderate. Not only the molar teeth, but even the jaw-bone
itself was thrown off." [p. 288].)

4. Prinz states that belief in the worm theory was shared by most
"civilized" nations of the past and by many "uncivilized races
even at present."
    Dental caries means hollow tooth, is called mushi-ha (room-
tooth) by Japanese, chung choo by Chinese. Tooth worm still
plays a part in oriental medicine, especially among countryside
inhabitants of Asia Minor, China, Japan, etc. [p. 16]
    In ancient India (4000-3000 BC) the tooth worm was thought to
cause dental caries (krimi-danta)
    About 41AD, Scribonius Largus, physician to Emperor Claudius,
claimed that worms cause dental caries. [p. 25]
    An ancient collection of manuscripts from the 13th century
referred to toothworms and prescribed remedies; these were

published in 1864 by Thomas O. Cockayne of London. [p. 34]

As late as 1540, the celebrated surgeon Ambroise Paré was a strong believer in worms.

In 1635 Jacques Houllier expressed the view that worms were not the cause of decayed teeth.

In 1757 Jacob Christian Schaeffer wrote "The Fancied Worms in Teeth", which disproved the presence of worms in decayed teeth.

In 1915, Dr. Gordon (formerly of U. of Penn.) related that Kukchi Indians of Guatemala called toothache "xulhe", meaning "mouth maggot". [p. 69]

5.   Pierre Fauchard ("Father of Dentistry") is generally credited with having had the greatest influence in arguing against the tooth worm. On the one hand he refers to "caries which gnaws as if a worm is eating the tooth" as "that which advances rapidly. It is the most to be feared and the most difficult to cure."[p. 44] But beyond this cute analogy, he is inclined not to accept the belief by "the vulgar and even certain authors ... that toothache and caries are caused by worms." Fauchard claims to have searched with excellent microscopes to no avail, further noting that teeth decayed from internal causes tend to argue against invasion by worms. But he does not rule out their possibility in some cases. [p. 55-6]

Section 7.   Pierre Fauchard, Father of Dentistry

   Discussion of Pierre Fauchard's, "The Surgeon Dentist or Treatise on the Teeth, In which is seen the means used to keep them clean and healthy, of beautifying them, of repairing their loss and remedies for their diseases and those of the gums and for accidents which may befall the other parts in their vicinity"

Translated from the Second Edition 1746 by Lillian Lindsay, 1946:

   In this definitive work, Fauchard has provided a summation of knowledge of dentistry as of the early 18th Century. Hermann Prinz, in his 1945 Dental Chronology (Lea & Febiger, Phila., p. 12) lamented: "It is very unfortunate that this book has never been translated into the English language. ... Undoubtedly it would have exercised a most profound and beneficial influence on the shaping of the destiny of the dental profession in Great Britain and in the U.S. A German translation ... appeared in Berlin in 1733. ... Fauchard is credited with having introduced the term 'dental caries' into dental terminology."
   A year later this translation was produced. Therefore, many or even most of those involved in the dialogue of the 30s and 40s concerning the proper nature of dentistry never read the Fauchard work. Thus, what we learn today of this work tends to be several steps removed from early partial translations. This explains why it seems to be still thought that lead was the filling of choice in Fauchard's time, whereas as discussed below this was not the case.
   Some of the most interesting aspects of this work from this writer's perspective are discussed and/or excerpted below. In particular, a few striking items are worthy of pre-summation:

1. Fauchard was much less inclined to retain a bothersome tooth than our contemporaries.

2. He repeatedly mentioned waiting for weeks or even months before filling a tooth after the caries had been removed.

3. While it is commonly thought that the practice in France at the time was to use lead for fillings, Fauchard clearly states his preference for tin, and clearly indicates that when he says lead he means tin or lead, or gold if preferred by the patient.

4. Fauchard regards the tooth to be a bone; the enamel is specifically characterized as analogous to a fingernail or horn.

5. Fauchard argues persuasively against the worm hypothesis; his work marks a definite turning point in popular conception.

6. Fauchard is nearly livid in his opposition to mercury anywhere on the human body (he does not specifically refer to mercury in the teeth; apparently this abortion was a later

invention. See page 3 below: ADDED NOTES ON ORIGIN OF MERCURY
AMALGAM IN 19TH CENTURY).

    Following are notes on Fauchard's work. Emphasis is on Volume
I, which concerned pathology, etc., and on that part of Vol. II,
which dealt with the filling of teeth. These notes are by no
means comprehensive, but may serve as an initial introduction and
guide.
Subjects covered:

TEETH ARE BONES
ENAMEL IS ATTACHED LIKE NAILS OR HORNS
WISDOM TEETH MAY CAUSE ABSCESS, TWITCHING
TEETHING AND DISEASE
ENEMIES OF THE TEETH
MERCURY - THE "GREATEST ENEMY" OF THE TEETH
ADDED NOTES ON ORIGIN OF MERCURY AMALGAM IN 19TH CENTURY
DISEASES CAUSED BY THE TEETH
TOOTHWORM HYPOTHESIS DISPUTED
CARIES
AUTOTHERAPY WITH URINE, FOR TOOTHACHE
ENGORGEMENTS IN CAPILLARIES OF THE GUMS
OPENING THE CANAL
WAIT WEEKS OR MONTHS BEFORE FILLING
MOLARS AND JAWBONE INFECTIONS
HEADACHE AND EARACHE CAUSED BY TEETH
LEAD MEANS TIN PREFERABLY, OR TIN OR LEAD, OR GOLD
ADDED NOTES ON ORIGIN OF FILLINGS IN TOOTH
DEEP CARIES WITH PAIN: PULL THE TOOTH, OR ?

Preface
    vii: "The teeth ... are the most polished and hardest of all
the bones of the human body but at the same time they are the
most subject to diseases which cause acute pain, and sometimes
become very dangerous. As the diversity of diseases, the causes
which they produce and their symptoms are infinite, the
operations which surgery has devised for their cure demand as
much variety of knowledge. ... "

TEETH ARE BONES; ENAMEL IS ATTACHED LIKE NAILS OR HORNS

    p. 1 "Teeth considered in their natural condition are the
whitest, hardest, and most compact bones of the human body.:

    p. 45 Fauchard discussed how displacements of bones and teeth
are of the same nature, thus, "When the tooth is loosened, it is
an incipient luxation."

    p. 9 Fauchard quotes M. de la Hire, mathematician and member
of the Royal Academy of Sciences, Memoires of the Academy 1699.
Examination of enamel under a microscope reveals "'that it is
composed of an infinity of little filaments, which are attached

on the inside of the tooth by their roots, almost like the nails and the horns are to the parts where they are attached. ...

"M. de la Hire is persuaded that the growth of these filaments takes place like the nails."

Fauchard relates de la Hire's observation that these filaments may be in bundles, particularly in the base of molars where separation of bundles can be seen. "'If the end of the filaments wear away little by little the separation of the two bundles will increase sufficiently to receive some hard parts of the food; and then there will be a little aperture on the base of the tooth. The interior part of the tooth is opened up and consequently the tooth will be lost.'"

p. 9-10 (cont) Fauchard disagrees, based on observations of older persons with enamel worn down.

p. 10: "I assert, nevertheless, that the fibres of the enamel once worn away are never replaced ... ."

Fauchard relates how layers of tooth form from the outside inward, and "that the enamel of the teeth is the first to be formed and that the number of layers increases the volume of the tooth..."

WISDOM TEETH MAY CAUSE ABSCESS, TWITCHING

p. 12 Regarding wisdom teeth, "... I have observed that these last molars, when they are cut at a late age cause sometimes fluxions and even an abscess in the neighboring parts; that can only produce twitching of the fleshy fibres of the gum which the crown of the tooth forces asunder in escaping in this way from its socket."

TEETHING AND DISEASE

p. 16ff Fauchard relates cutting of milk teeth to diseases of children, including pain of eyes and face, coughs, fever, diarrhoea, nausea, vomiting, convulsions, terror, lethargy, and sometimes death.

ENEMIES OF THE TEETH

p. 37-8 Fauchard discusses causes of diseases of teeth, including external causes. These include bits of food which stick to teeth or gums, cold and heat, inclement weather which causes colds etc., breaking or loosening of teeth, abrading of enamel in an attempt to clean it, too much tobacco, falls and violent blows, negligence and lack of care in keeping them clean.

MERCURY - THE "GREATEST ENEMY" OF THE TEETH

Fauchard was nearly livid in his opposition to mercury anywhere in contact with the human body. (He did not specifically refer to mercury in the teeth; apparently this was a later invention -- a hundred years later! Fillings of a paste-mixture, or "amalgam", of mercury and coin-silver were reportedly first used in about 1819 by Tavenu in France and Bell in England. [Source: T. Wilwerding, C.J. Vacanti, History of Dentistry, 1997-8, Creighton U.])

   In his definitive work, "The Surgeon-Dentist ...", p. 38-9 Fauchard asserted that "Their [the teeth's] greatest enemy is mercury, vulgarly called quick-silver. Not only in itself but by the bad effects which it produces in the system, by corrosives with which preparations of mercury are mixed, or by the combinations it makes in our bodies with different principles by long retention, particularly when it is not properly excreted. The effects of mercury are swelling of the gums which it corrodes and destroys; it acts in the same way on the membrane which lines the roots of the teeth, either internally or externally, it desiccates them so to speak ... and makes them fall out or destroys them by the caries to which it gives rise. These bad effects are seen only too often, especially the bad effect of mercury when taken by people who do not know how to use it. Physicians and surgeons who have the most experience in venereal diseases, although they prescribe it with great caution, have difficulty enough in preventing the destruction of the teeth even with all the skill and industry of which they are capable. Gilders of ormolu, makers of mirrors, plumbers, and all those who work in the mines are only too often the victims of the bad effects of mercury, particularly on their teeth."

ADDED NOTES ON ORIGIN OF MERCURY AMALGAM IN 19TH CENTURY

   [Fillings of a paste-mixture (amalgam) of mercury and coin-silver was used as early as 1819 by Tavenu in France and Bell in England. (Source: T. Wilwerding, C.J. Vacanti, History of Dentistry, 1997-8, Creighton U.) The use of this "amalgam" of silver and mercury by the Crawkours sparked the Amalgam War of the mid 1800s, as (a) any substance with mercury was opposed by the American Society of Dental Surgeons and (2) mercury with pure silver expanded. G.V. Black's alloys of tin-silver (plus small quantities of copper and zinc as per subsequent ADA guidelines), amalgamated with mercury, solved the expansion problem, but did not address the mercury problem. Black's and subsequent amalgams contain nearly half, approx. 45%, mercury. (per G.V. Black, Vol. 2, 1936; Syllabus, History of Dentistry, A.I. Coleman, 1971); see also Section 8.b., "Black on Mercury", below.]

DISEASES CAUSED BY THE TEETH

   p. 43 Diseases caused by the teeth are listed, including abortion, nausea, vomiting, diarrhhoea, fever, insomnia, delirium, headache, emaciation (of infants), convulsions, ptyalism, ulcer of parotid and tonsils, earaches and ear infections, ophthalmia or inflammation of eyes, tumors of cheek, polypus, lachrymal fistulae.

TOOTHWORM HYPOTHESIS DISPUTED

Pierre Fauchard ("Father of Dentistry") is generally credited with having had the greatest influence in arguing against the tooth worm. On the one hand he refers to "caries which gnaws as if a worm is eating the tooth" as "that which advances rapidly. It is the most to be feared and the most difficult to cure."[p. 44] But beyond this cute analogy, he is inclined not to accept the belief by "the vulgar and even certain authors ... that toothache and caries are caused by worms." Fauchard claims to have searched with excellent microscopes to no avail, further noting that teeth decayed from internal causes tend to argue against invasion by worms. But he does not rule out their possibility in some cases. [p. 55-6]

CARIES

p. 45 Fauchard notes that the "ravages of caries are greatest from 25 to 50 years of age."

FILLINGS - WAIT DAYS OR MONTHS TO FILL; SOME IMPOSSIBLE

p. 60 "When a tooth is slightly carious it is enough to remove the caries by instruments, of which I shall speak presently, and to fill the cavity with lead. [Note, as discussed later, that Fauchard means tin, lead or gold when saying lead] When the caries penetrates further and causes pain after removal, put into the cavity every day a ball of cotton dipped in oil of cinnamon or cloves. ... Four or five days later remove the carious matter left in the cavity. ... If after enough time has elapsed the pain does not cease, the actual cautery must be applied and several months later fill the cavity if the condition of the carious cavity permits, because sometimes there are cavities which it is impossible to fill.

"When the caries penetrates into the cavity of the tooth it may start an abscess there. ... I introduced the point of my probe into the caries up to the cavity of the tooth to evacuate the matter. From the moment the pus was evacuated, the pain ceased. I leave such people alone for 2 or 3 months. At the end of this time I fill the teeth to prevent further decay."

AUTOTHERAPY WITH URINE, FOR TOOTHACHE
ENGORGEMENTS FORM AT THE ENDS OF THE CAPILLARIES OF THE GUMS

p. 61-2 Fauchard provides details of two topical remedies for toothache, and then discusses urine.

"I have relieved many people by the following remedy when nearly all the teeth were carious and when toothache was always a torment.

"It consists of rinsing the mouth every morning and even in the evening before going to bed with several spoonfuls of the patient's urine freshly made, presuming it is healthy. ...

"To convince as to the virtue of urine, it suffices to know that it is composed of a serous liquor impregnated with a volatile salt and some oil. These active substances give it many qualities which make it [p. 62] appropriate for diseases. Experience teaches us that the urine of a healthy person assuages and calms the pain of gout, and removes obstructions, etc. It is thus a resolutive which can dissipate engorgements which form at the ends of the capillaries of the gums and the tumours which rise in the mouth and may prevent and destroy by degrees many troubles which arise there."

OPENING THE CANAL -- WAIT WEEKS OR MONTHS BEFORE FILLING

P. 63, Chapter 10: Trepanning the teeth when they are worn down or carious and cause toothache

In the case of toothaches in incisors and canines, herein Fauchard discusses first removing carious matter and then opening the canal with a reamer -- either a sewing needle, "minikin" pin, or drill (in the case of a canal too narrow for needle or pin).

p. 64 "After this operation some weeks must elapse without attempting any more with the tooth, and to prevent any further decay a ball of cotton dipped in a little oil of cinnamon with cloves must be put in the cavity. This must be left for several months [note reference to months again] taking care to remove the cotton from time to time. Care must be taken to do this gently without compression so that any matter which happens to be there may escape through the cotton which is only put there to keep out the food and prevent further decay. If the cotton is made tight at first so that the matter cannot escape it will thicken and congest and may cause much pain, if the nervous part of the tooth be not already dried up or destroyed. The same happens after plugging the tooth, which will make it necessary to remove it and allow discharge for a considerable time before putting it back."

MOLARS AND JAWBONE INFECTIONS

Fauchard notes that the situation is more difficult with molars, which have several roots, so "it is not possible to operate with great exactitude. Henard advises that these teeth must be drawn, or at least to decapitate them. ... [p. 65] he has seen a good deal of abscess inside teeth without any external decay, and that after having fractured them, he found purulent matter of an insupportable odour which ... had putrified in the tooth ... . It must not be thought that it is only this part which suffers, but it can be judged that the surrounding parts would be greatly irritated and intensely painful. ... [The ill effects] end as a rule in an abscess and fistulae in the gums and surrounding parts ... "

HEADACHE AND EARACHE CAUSED BY TEETH

Chapter XXXIII, p. 154, "Four observations on violent pains in the head caused by the teeth" -- Fauchard reports on violent earaches and headaches cured by the removal of (often symptomless) carious teeth.

Volume II

LEAD MEANS TIN PREFERABLY, OR TIN OR LEAD, OR GOLD

p. 27 "Although I use the word lead often for filling hollow and carious teeth, finely beaten tin is to be preferred." This is "because lead blackens and does not last so long. both [tin and lead] are preferable to gold for filling carious cavities in teeth because they are lighter than gold, are pliable and adapt themselves better. ... Besides gold is dear [costly] ... ."

ADDED NOTES ON ORIGIN OF FILLINGS IN TOOTH

[It is noted that the first filling of teeth with lead was apparently by Celsus in 30 AD to enable extraction without fracturing the crown, not for preservation of the tooth. Gold foil was used for filling (preserving) teeth as early as 1514 AD by Giovanni da Vigo. (Source: T. Wilwerding, C.J. Vacanti, History of Dentistry, 1997-8, Creighton U.)]

DEEP CARIES WITH PAIN: PULL THE TOOTH, OR ?

p. 30 Fauchard offers if "the pain starts afresh or persists, if also one is assured of the depth of the caries there is no other way [but] to draw the tooth ... .
Fauchard further notes that it is not always possible to avoid exposing the nerve, so that the tooth must be cauterized with a brass knitting needle or other instrument, and covered or filled with cotton steeped in oil of cinnamon "... until time has been gained for filling it".

Section 8.   G.V. Black

a.   "The Dentist's Opportunity"
[from G.V. Black, pp. 398-410, "Systemic Effects of Chronic
Infections of the Mouth", in Special Dental Pathology, 1915]
    Herein Black refers to and enthusiastically endorses the
recent works of Hunter, Billings, Rosenow and others on the
subject. The timing of this publication, coming in the last year
of G.V. Black's lifetime (Son A.D. continued to publish it as
Vol. 4 of collected works), was such that the full implications
of Rosenow's most recent (1914) work was as yet not fully clear.
 Black cites (1) Rosenow's 1914 qualification of earlier vaccine
results and (2) Rosenow's 1914 works on transmutation and new
culture methodology, which latter items would come to fully
explain and overcome the need for qualification.
    Rosenow had said vaccines for arthritis may not have worked
well because the were made from oral foci organisms, which may
have been different in character from those in the lesion at the
time; Rosenow's works on transmutation and culture methodology
would show them to be the same organism altered by conditions,
and he would be now begin to be able to culture it successfully
from any location with proper methodology -- which methodology
Rosenow would continue to use successfully through 1958. Black,
not around for follow-up verification, did not fully pick up on
Rosenow's early indication that this was the case, and hence
Black wrote that the organism in the focus and that in the
secondary lesion were different organisms; however, he did leave
open the possibility that the morphology of the primary organism
may have changed and caused the secondary lesion.
    Black vehemently called for "the eradication of the foci for
the protection of the health of all persons, whether apparently
suffering or not." It is unfortunate that Black was not fully
beneficiary to the fact that all compromised teeth are foci, or
it can be assumed he would have made this known to the dental
community. (It is noted that G.V.'s son A.D. Black published in
the same year, 1915, a definitive review of knowledge from the
previous century concerning the relation between oral infections
and diseases of the eye.) In any case, G.V. accepted that
organisms from oral foci enter the circulation and locate in
particular tissues, and that these are in some way responsible
for secondary effects including most frequently arthritis,
endocarditis, nephritis, cholecystitis, stomach ulcers and
appendicitis, and/or general impairment of health and vigor.
    Black characterized the situation as "The Dentist's
Opportunity: The opportunity before the dental profession to
take an important part in the preservation of the general health
is almost without parallel in medical advancement. ...
Eradication of mouth foci should not be delayed until secondary
effects have become manifest. Every dentist, who has a full
appreciation of the situation, will realize that, in the
management of cases, he is doing his highest duty to humanity in
the preservation of health by keeping the mouths under his care

free from these centers of distribution of infection."

b. G.V. Black on Mercury

G.V. Black died in 1915, but his various works continued to be published long afterwards. Thus, Vol. 2 of the 1936 four-volume edition of his work blamed charlatan operators for the negative reaction against amalgam which had precipitated the amalgam war in the mid-19th Century, but does not mention other objections that had been raised against mercury. Rather, the volume states that it is assumed that the material used [by the Crawkours] was pure silver and mercury, which "soon led to the mixing of shavings of silver coins with mercury [which] would set very slowly, and show considerable expansion."

Whereas, Coleman's Syllabus, p. 77, quotes the American Society of Dental Surgeons, in the mid-19th Century, as having stated that "the use of Lithodeon mineral paste, and all other substances of which mercury is an ingredient, is injurious to the teeth...." The American Society of Dental Surgeons had unanimously condemned its use, whereas an upstart association of Dentists, the American Dental Association, supported the use of mercury in tooth fillings. The former was disbanded in the mid-19th Century, whereas the latter continues to serve as the primary association of dentists to this day.

Black's own particular contribution involved experimentation with various alloys in place of pure silver, which alloys when mixed with mercury would not change bulk while or after hardening. Black discovered the principle of annealing, whereby a silver-tin alloy (65-35) melted in a closed electric crucible in presence of hydrogen, would neither expand nor contract when amalgamated [with mercury] on the same day. He also found that purities of different batches of metals were not consistent. He determined that "Therefore, no fixed formula could be good for general use." In general it was found that annealed alloys of <70% silver would shrink and >75% silver would expand.

A table is presented with various portions of silver, from 40% to 75%, with the remainder tin. The table also lists various "percent of mercury" values added, which varied from a low of 32.13 to a high of 55%; average value 45.5%. Also listed (p. 13) are average relative composition of other components (without reference to mercury) specified by ADA Specification No. 1: silver 65% min., copper 6% max., Zinc 2% max., Tin 25% min.

Black is thus credited with having developed "balanced amalgam alloys" (cudental.creighton.edu/htm/history.htm); more correctly this would be referred to as balanced alloys for amalgams, i.e. amalgamization with mercury. The balance refers to those metals excluding mercury, which balance minimizes volume change. This "balance" would thus eliminate the problem of expansion that would occur with pure silver when amalgamated with mercury, but would do nothing to ameliorate the basic problem with mercury toxicity -- amalgamization does not lock in the mercury and prohibit it from acting as the poison it is.

Section 9.   General PhD Criteria - Issues and Responses

In that the AABD is a non-resident, non-conventional post-graduate institution, it is recognized that particular care need be taken to assure that the level of bona-fide study effort underlying a petition for the award of a PhD degree substantively satisfies customary conventional criteria, both quantitatively and qualitatively. Further, insofar as the AABD is primarily involved with education at the post-doctoral level (CME), a petitioner to the AABD for the PhD degree may expect to be held to a correspondingly higher level.

The Encyclopedia Britannica gives the following description of the PhD, which may serve as a useful guideline:
    "The minimum period of study accepted for the degree of PhD is two years after obtaining a bachelor's degree; but in practice, three, and even four years of study are found necessary. In addition to carrying on an investigation in the field of his main subject of study, the candidate for the degree of Ph. D. is usually required to pass examinations on one or two subordinate subjects, to possess a reading knowledge of French and German ... and to submit -- usually in printed form -- the dissertation which embodies the results of his researches."

Issue 1.1 (Time Period):
    Satisfaction of minimum quantitative level of effort may properly be assessed through consideration of any combination of verifiable conventional or independent study. Given the professional nature of research work meriting consideration for recognition by the AABD, much of which may be in advance of the establishment of conventional programs of study, the AABD is clearly authorized to grant up to full time-credit for either or any combination of (a) satisfactory completion of courses of historical study at the graduate level in an accredited university program, and/or (b) verifiable independent study.

Response 1.1:
    The research effort underlying this petition was conducted over the period 1988 through 1999, involving a minimum of 50% level of full-time effort, or a minimum of 5.5 man-years effort. Written evidence of this level of effort is provided in compilations previously submitted, i.e., as primarily but not exclusively presented in reports bearing titles of *AUTOHEMOTHERAPY REFERENCE MANUAL* and *REFERENCE MANUAL ROSENOW ET AL*, in this dissertation, *MEDICINE'S GRANDEST FRAUD PHD*, in the study and compilation of approximately 100 articles authored by E.C.Rosenow (copy provided to the AABD in March 1999), and various other materials provided to the AABD and/or associates over the past two years. Supplementary evidence is provided at www.InstituteOfScience.com.
    Associated research efforts involving extensive indirectly-related theoretical/historical physical-chemical studies were

conducted primarily over the period 1981 through 1988, involving a minimum of 50% level of full-time effort during this period, or a minimum of 3.5 man-years effort (plus additional part-time efforts through 1999). Written evidence of this level of effort is provided on the internet at www.Hydration.com.

These above time estimates are conservative, as evidenced by above-cited written materials.

Additionally, prior to withdrawal due to temporary assignment to Vietnam with the U.S. Department of State, the petitioner had satisfactorily completed a year of graduate study as a direct to PhD and honor student (elected to Pi Sigma Alpha Honor Society) in historical studies at the Georgetown University Graduate School, which record of study satisfied U.S. Department of State (Agency for International Development) requirements relative to assignment of government service grade level.

While serving with the U.S. State Department, the petitioner was able to develop analytical skills indispensable to initiating the unique research scope associated with this petition, for which efforts he received a Meritorious Service award. Further, justification for consideration of this independent effort in lieu of accredited coursework rests on the fact that accredited coursework in the areas herein addressed is not currently available. Indeed in part the purpose of this petition is to establish a foundation(s) for such studies in the future.

Issue 1.2 (Subordinate Subjects):

On the question of documentation of "one or two subordinate subjects" as discussed by Encyclopedia Britannica, the intent is to assure that the petitioner has attained a grasp of subordinate or otherwise related disciplines, and/or the process of historical research, so as to enable extension into future research and/or teaching efforts as appropriate. Accordingly, examination of such capability may be comprised of review of written essay materials, in lieu of formal examinations. In cases of independent study, without prior precedents of on-going courses of instruction, such a substitution of written essay materials may in fact be not merely optional but rather required due to the non-existence of alternate testing methodology.

Response 1.2:

Evidence of satisfactory completion of study in three augmentative historical subject areas, (a) focal infection, (b) autohemotherapy, and (c) physical science considerations, is to be found in previously submitted (a) *REFERENCE MANUAL ROSENOW ET AL*, an Introduction to *Focal Infection* by Frank Billings, and Introduction to *The Dental-Mental Connection* (a compilation of works of H. Cotton and H. Upson), and (b) the *AUTOHEMOTHERAPY REFERENCE MANUAL*; and (c) at Hydration.com and *Nature* 338, 456, resp.

Issue 1.3 (Language Requirement):

The ability to translate (for the purpose of reading comprehension) critical portions of technical articles from German, in particular relative to these areas of study, is very useful due to the nature of the historical literature.

Response 1.3:
   The German language requirement was satisfied Oct. 21, 1965 by formal examination at Georgetown University Graduate School. In addition, portions of articles translated from German, French and Italian technical literature were submitted as examples of the practical utility of this language requirement and its fulfillment.

Issue 1.4 (Qualitative Level of Effort):
   Satisfaction of minimum qualitative level of effort, taken as a given to generally involve substantive issues of relevance and potential consequence within the field, is customarily and predominantly determined by the written dissertation, which may additionally be supported by oral (essay) examination (or "dissertation defense"). Such oral dissertation defense may be of varying length, so long as it (a) clearly authenticates authorship of the dissertation, (b) establishes that the petitioner is capable of defense of the dissertation, particularly including its most potentially controversial aspects, and (c) demonstrates that the petitioner is capable of commencing with lecturing on the college level.
   Again, it is acknowledged that any AABD-sanctioned PhD petitioner must be held to a higher level, insofar as students are themselves likely to be holders of doctoral degrees.
   Accordingly, an AABD-associated research effort aspiring to PhD recognition must be regarded as involving substantive issues of demonstrated essential interest to professionals in the field.
 Satisfaction of this condition may properly be assessed through consideration of evidence of any combination of post-doctoral level professional presentations, consultations and/or publications.

Response 1.4:
   As evidence of minimally-satisfactory level of qualitative effort at the post-doctoral level, kind consideration is requested of: (a) presentations to the AABD at annual meetings in 1998 and 1999, and to the Capital University of (Graduate) Integrative Medicine (CUIN) in 1998; and participation as speaker (with Dr. David Kennedy, DDS, former President of the IAOMT) on Holistic Dentistry Panel at Los Angeles Convention Center, Oct. 1998; and with Drs. Kennedy, DDS, and Hans Gruen, MD, on the Awareness 2000 health panel in 1999; (b) consultations with Dr. Arana of the AABD (numerous); Dr. Lowell Weiner, Dean of Dentistry, CUIN, in 1997 (extensive); Dr. George Meinig (numerous and extensive); Dr. Christopher J. Hussar (numerous and extensive); various dental and legal professionals on referral/request of the AABD; and 1999 AABD-follow-up

correspondence with Drs. Hussar, Haley, Bouquot, Klinghardt and Arana (relevant portions have been incorporated above); and (c) publication in Nature, London (Vol. 338, p. 456, 1989), on history of science considerations related to above-cited theoretical, indirectly-related studies. In particular, presentations at 1998 and 1999 AABD meetings, associated participation in related Q. and A. sessions, and follow-up as incorporated herein are proposed as having in large measure satisfied requirements for defense (examination) of doctoral dissertation. Additionally the petitioner would be pleased to provide further documentation in response to any specific requests of the faculty and/or further elaboration on any questions or issues discussed elsewhere in this presentation.

Issue 1.5:
   Main dissertation components, as set forth by Turabian, are: Title Page, Preface, Table of contents, List of Tables/ Illustrations, Introduction, Body, Appendices, Bibliography. There is flexibility to this format, as such matters "must be left to the good sense of the writer".

Response 1.5:
   The PhD dissertation incorporates all essential components of the indicated format.

BIBLIOGRAPHY (partial; ALSO see particularly JADA Chronology)

Appleton, J.L.T., Jr., *Bacterial Infection*, Lea & Febiger, Philadelphia 1933, 565-577.

Atkinson, Donald T., *Magic, Myth and Medicine*, World Publishing Co., Cleveland and New York, 1956 (on the history of dentistry).

Austin, Louie T., D.D.S., and Thomas J. Cook, D.D.S., "Bacteriologic Study of Normal Vital Teeth", *J.A.D.A.* 16: 894-6 (May) 1929

Austin, Louie T., DDS, Rochester, Minn., "Relationship of Dental Sepsis to Systemic Disease", *J.A.D.A.*, 27, May 1940, 684-688.

Beeson, PB and W McDermott, *Cecil Loeb Textbook of Medicine*, W.B. Saunders, Phila. and London, 1963, p. 1479.

Beeson, Paul B., in Bowers, J. & E. Purcell, eds., *Advances in American Medicine: Essays at the Bicentennial*, 1, (N. Y., J. Macy Found. 1976), 151-2, "Focal Infection and Systemic Disease"

Bellizzi, R and WP Cruse, *J. of Endodontics* Vol. 6 (May 1980), 576-580, "A historic review of endodontics, 1689-1963, part 3".

Bierring, Walter L., "Focal Infection: Quarter Century Survey", *JAMA* 111 (Oct. 29, 1938), 1623-1627.

Billings, Frank, *Arch. Int. Med.* April 1912, 484-498, "Chronic Focal Infections & Etiologic Relations to Arthritis & Nephritis".

Billings, Frank, [JAMA 1922;78:1097-1105]

Bremner, M. D. K., DDS, FACD; The Story of Dentistry, Rev. 3rd Ed., Dental Items of Interest Publ. Co., Brooklyn 1954, p. 90-91

Burket, Lester W., *Oral Medicine* 6th Ed., J.B. Lippincott Co., Phila., 1971, 550-556.

Chase, A., *Magic Shots*, 1980, 424-431.

Coleman, A. I.; *A Syllabus - History of Dentistry*

Coolidge, E. D., *JADA* 61 (1960) 676-688, "Past and present concepts in endodontics"

Crowley, M.C., *Am. J. Orthodontics* (Oral Surg. Sect.) 32, 126-130, Feb. 1946.

DiStefano, P.G., *Annali di Stomatol.* (Rome) 20 (1971), 243-254.

Easlick, Kenneth A., *Jour. Am. Dent. Assn.* 42 (1951), 619-632.

Easlick KA, *JADA* 46 (Feb. 1953), 179-183, "The role of the pulpless tooth in systemic disease: a summary".

Fauchard, Pierre; *The Surgeon Dentist*, 1746; Translation by Lilian Lindsay, Butterworth & Co., 1946

Fischer, Martin H.; *Dental Summary*, August 1915, Vol. 35, 607, from an address to the Cincinnati Dental Society, Jan. 29, 1915, 613-622, 716-734.

Fishbein, Morris, *The American Medical Association 1847 to 1947*, 1947, Philadelphia, W.B. Saunders

Grossman, Louis I., *Root Canal Therapy*, 1940, 15-26; 1946, 154-172.

Grossman, Louis I., *Oral Surg., Oral Med., Oral Path.*,13, 1130-1133, "Evaluation of a Method to Determine the Presence of a Focus of Infection", 1960

Grossman, Louis I., *JADA* 93 (July 1976), 78-87, "Endodontics 1776-1996"; refers to L. I. Grossman's *Root Canal Therapy*, 1940, and its new title *Endodontic Practice*, 1974.

Grossman, L.I., *Endodontic Practice*, 10th Ed, Lea & Febiger 1981

Grossman, Louis I., Seymour Oliet and Carlos E. Del Rio, *Endodontic Practice*, Eleventh Edition, Lea & Febiger, Philadelphia, 1988, p. 234-240.

Haden, Russell, L., *Dental Infection and Systemic Disease*, Lea and Febiger, Philadelphia, Pa., U.S.A. 1928, p.159

Henrici, Arthur T. and Thomas B. and Hartzell, "The Bacteriology of Vital Pulps" , *J. Dent. Research* 1:419-422 (Dec.) 1919

Hirsch, Edwin F., *Frank Billings, The Architect of Medical Education, An Apostle of Excellence in Medical Practice; A Leader in Chicago Medicine*, University of Chicago, 1966.

Holman, W.L., "Focal Infection and 'Elective Localization', A Critical Review", *Archives Path & Lab. Med.* 5 1928, 68-136; 133.

Holman, W.L., "The Localization in Animals of Bacteria Isolated from Foci of Infection", *JAMA* 88 (Feb. 5, 1927), 424-5.

Howe, Percy R., THE DENTAL COSMOS, LXI (1919), Part 1, 33-40, "To What Degree are Oral Pathological Conditions Responsible for Systemic Disease?"

Hughes RA, *British Journal of Rheumatology* 33 (1994), 370-7, "Focal Infection Revisited".

Huxtable, H.S. and Batterson, G.E.; *Summary Suggestion guide on teaching Dental History*, American Academy of History of Dentistry, 1966

Ingle, John I., *Endodontics*, Third Edition, Lea and Febiger, Philadelphia, 1985, p. 1.

JAMA 150 (Oct. 4, 1952), Editorial: "Focal Infection", 490-1.

Jawetz, E., *Oral Surg., Oral Med., Oral Path.* 8 (1955), 1063, "The Rise and Fall of Focal Infection".

Jawetz, E., *Oral Surg., Oral Med., Oral Path.* 8 (1955), 1069-1073, "Virus infections of interest to the dentist"

Kanner, Leo; Folklore of the Teeth, MacMillan, NY, 1928, p. 107.

Kern, Richard A., "What is left of the theory of focal infection?", *M. Clin. North America* 34 (Nov. 1952): 1705-1712. "a boil on the back of the neck is at times followed by a perinephritic abscess.

Kolmer, J.A., "Focal infection in relation to health and disease", *A.D.A. Journal* 45:139-159, August 14, 1 (1940).

Lindsay, Lilian; Short History of Dentistry, Bale & Sons, London 1933

MacNevin, M.G. and Vaughn, H.S., *Mouth Infections and Their Relation to Systemic Disease*, New York, Joseph Purcell Research Memorial, 1930, 78-91.

Maggio, Joseph, *Prevention* 41, October 1989 [President, AAE]

Miller, Neil R., *Walsh and Hoyt's Clinical Neuro-Ophthalmology* Fourth Edition, Williams and Wilkins 1982: Baltimore/London.

Miller, W. D.; *Dental Cosmos*, 1891, 33, 689

Morse, D. R., *Oral Surg.* 43 (March 1977), 436-451, "Immunologic Aspects of pulpal-periapical diseases."

Morse, D. R., in Cohen, S. and R. C. Burns, Pathways of the Pulp, C.V. Mosby, St. Louis, 1987, p. 378

Navazesh M and R Mulligan, Special Care in Dentistry, 1995, Jan-Feb, 15(1): 11-9.

Newman, H.N., J. of Dental Research 71(11), Nov., 1992, p. 1854, and Periodontal Abstracts Volume 41 Number 3, 1993, 73-77

Nickel AC and AR Hufford, *Arch. Int. Med.*41 (1928), 210-230, "Elective Localization of Streptococci Isolated from Cases of Peptic Ulcer", p. 215 [1928]

Norton, Alan, *The New Dimensions of Medicine*, Hodder and Stroughton, London 1969]

Okell, C.C., and S.D. Elliot, *The Lancet* CCXXIX (Oct. 19, 1935), 869-872, "Bacteriaemia and oral sepsis, with special reference to the aetiology of subacute endocarditis"

Price, Weston, *Dental Infection, Oral and Systemic*, 1923: Cleveland, Penton Pub. Co.

Prinz, Hermann; *Dental Chronology*, Febiger, Phila., 1945Fish, E.W. and I. MacLean, "The Distribution of Oral Streptococci in the Tissues", *British Dental Journal* 61 (1936), 336-362.

Reimann, Hobart A., and Havens, W. Paul, *J.A.M.A.*, 114, 1 (1940), "Focal Infection and Systemic Disease: A Critical Appraisal".

Reines, Brandon P., *Science* 245 (Aug. 11, 1989), Letters, refers to Paul Beeson as "the doyen of American internal medicine"

Rhein ML, F. Krasnow and WJ Gies, *Dental Cosmos* lxviii (Oct. 1926), 971-981, "A Prolonged Study of the Electrolytic Treatment of Dental Focal Infection - A Preliminary Report", p. 970

Rhoads, P.S. and G.F. Dick, *JADA* 19 (November 1932), 1844-1893, "Roentgenographically negative pulpless teeth as foci of infection: Results of quantitative cultures"

Rosenow, E. C., J.A.M.A. LXV 1688 (1915).

Rosenow, E.C., Jour. Lab. and Clin. Med. 14:504-512, 1929, p. 506

Rosenow, E.C., Studies on focal infection, elective localization and cataphoretic velocity of streptococci. Dental Cosmos 76:721-744 (July) 1934; Brit. Jour. Dent. Sc. 79:175-183 (Oct.) 1934.

Rosenow, E.C., Isolation of bacteria from virus and phage by serial dilution, Arch. Path. 26: 70-76, July 1938

Rosenow, E. C., Dental Centenary Proceedings, Maryland State Dental Association and A.D.A., March 1940, p. 261-82.

Rosenow, E.C., Infection in filed, vital, roentgeno-graphically negative teeth, Cincinnati J. Med. 25: 329-339, Oct. 1944.

Rosenow, E.C., Streptococci in etiology of diverse diseases, including diseases of nervous system, J. Nerv. and Ment. Dis.

117: 415-428, May 1953.

Rosenow, E.C., J. Nerv. & Ment. Dis. 122: 238-247, 321-331 (1955)

Seltzer, S., in Cohen, S. and R. C. Burns, *Pathways of the Pulp*, C.V. Mosby, St. Louis, 1987, p 1.

Sharp, George C., *J.A.D.A. and Dental Cosmos*, 24 (August 1937), 1231-1242, "The historical and biological aspects of the pulpless tooth question".

Slocumb, Charles H., Melvin W. Binger, et al.: "Focal Infection", *JAMA* 117 (Dec. 20, 1941), 2161-2164.

Swanson, W.F. and L.E. Van Kirk, *J. Dent. Res.* 15 (Sept., 1936), 315: "Results of culturing 1800 pulpless teeth".

Thoden van Velzen, S.K., L. Abraham-Inpijn and W.R. Moorer, J. Clin. Periodont. 11 (1984) 209-220

Topazian, D.S., *Indian J. of Med. Sci.* 16 (1962), 1072-1083, "The present status of the theory of focal infection."

Tunnicliff, Ruth and Carolyn Hammond, "Presence of Bacteria in Pulps of Intact Teeth", *J.A.D.A. and Dental Cosmos* 24: 1663-1666 (Oct) 1937

Valentine Eugenia and Martha van Meter, *J. Infectious Disease* 47 (July 1930), 56-82, "The Localization of Streptococci in the Tissues of Rabbits."

White, Leon E. (1928): "The location of the focus in optic nerve disturbances from infection", *Ann. Otol. Rhinol. Laryngol.* 27 (1928), 128-164. [28Q3]

Wiene, Franklin S., *Endodontic Therapy*, C.V. Mosby Company, St. Louis 1989, 1-2.

Wilkie DPD, *Brit. Med. J.* 1 (1928), 481-4, "Some Aspects of Gall-Bladder Disease"

Wolfson, B.L., *Cal. State Dental Assoc.* 25 (1949), 106, "Endodontia and tooth conservation".

Woods, Alan C., *Am. J. Ophth.* 25 (Dec. 1942), 1423-1444, "Focal Infection"

AMERICAN ACADEMY OF BIOLOGICAL DENTISTRY

has conferred on STUART HALE SHAKMAN the degree

Doctor of Philosophy
in the History of Dentistry

with all the rights and privileges thereunto appertaining. In witness thereof this diploma is awarded by the AABD upon the recommendation of the faculty.

Christopher J. Hussar, DDS, DO, Faculty

Signed and sealed on this 7th day of July, 1999
Carmel, California

Edward M. Arana, DDS, President

www.ingramcontent.com/pod-product-compliance
Lightning Source LLC
Chambersburg PA
CBHW081116170526

45165CB00008B/2458